Navigating Life
with a Brain Tumor

Navigating Life with a Brain Tumor

Lynne P. Taylor, MD, FAAN

Associate Professor, Neuro-Oncology
Director of Palliative Care
Tufts Medical Center
Boston, MA

Alyx B. Porter Umphrey, MD

Assistant Professor of Neurology
Mayo Clinic
Scottsdale, AZ

Diane Richard

Minneapolis, MN

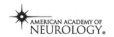

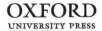

Oxford University Press is a department of the University of Oxford.
It furthers the University's objective of excellence in research, scholarship,
and education by publishing worldwide.

Oxford   New York
Auckland   Cape Town   Dar es Salaam   Hong Kong   Karachi
Kuala Lumpur   Madrid   Melbourne   Mexico City   Nairobi
New Delhi   Shanghai   Taipei   Toronto

With offices in
Argentina   Austria   Brazil   Chile   Czech Republic   France   Greece
Guatemala   Hungary   Italy   Japan   Poland   Portugal   Singapore
South Korea   Switzerland   Thailand   Turkey   Ukraine   Vietnam

Oxford is a registered trademark of Oxford University Press in
the UK and certain other countries.

Published in the United States of America by
Oxford University Press
198 Madison Avenue, New York, NY 10016

© American Academy of Neurology 2013

Library of Congress Cataloging-in-Publication Data

Taylor, Lynne P.
Navigating life with a brain tumor / Lynne P. Taylor, Alyx B. Porter Umphrey, Diane Richard.
p. cm.
Includes index.
ISBN 978-0-19-989779-7 (pbk.)
1. Brain—Tumors—Treatment. 2. Brain—Tumors—Popular works.
I. Porter Umphrey, Alyx B.   II. Richard, Diane, 1966-   III. Title.
RC280.B7T39 2013
616.99'481—dc23   2012011186

This material is not intended to be, and should not be considered, a substitute for medical or other professional
advice. Treatment for the conditions described in this material is highly dependent on the individual
circumstances. And, while this material is designed to offer accurate information with respect to the subject
matter covered and to be current as of the time it was written, research and knowledge about medical and health
issues is constantly evolving and dose schedules for medications are being revised continually, with new side
effects recognized and accounted for regularly. Readers must therefore always check the product information
and clinical procedures with the most up-to-date published product information and data sheets provided by
the manufacturers and the most recent codes of conduct and safety regulation. The publisher and the authors
make no representations or warranties to readers, express or implied, as to the accuracy or completeness of this
material. Without limiting the foregoing, the publisher and the authors make no representations or warranties as
to the accuracy or efficacy of the drug dosages mentioned in the material. The authors and the publisher do not
accept, and expressly disclaim, any responsibility for any liability, loss or risk that may be claimed or incurred as a
consequence of the use and/or application of any of the contents of this material.

Disclosure statements for potential conflicts of interest provided by the authors are available upon request
from the American Academy of Neurology, 201 Chicago Avenue, Minneapolis, MN 55415; Attn: *Neurology
Now Books*.

To protect the privacy of the patients mentioned herewith, we refer only to each patient's first name.
However, each case is real and no details, other than a shortening o f patient names, have been modified.

1 3 5 7 9 8 6 4 2
Printed in the United States of America on acid-free paper

This is dedicated to the brave patients who inspire us daily

and the people who love them

CONTENTS

About The AAN's *Neurology Now*™ Book Series | xi
   Lisa M. Shulman, MD
Preface | xv
   Lynne P. Taylor, MD
Acknowledgments | xvii

PART 1: Where Do I Begin?

Introduction | 3
   Step 1: Take a Deep Breath | 4
   Step 2: Seek Out Information | 4
   Step 3: Assemble Your Team | 6
   Step 4: Keep a Journal | 7

1: A Look Inside Your Brain | 8
   Basics About the Brain | 8
   Understanding Brain Tumors | 13
   A Search for Why | 20
   Getting a Diagnosis | 22

2: Diagnosis | 24

  Assessment and Plan | 25

  Getting the Medical Help You Need | 35

  Assembling Your Team | 37

  Finalizing Your Treatment Team | 41

  Understanding Your Prognosis | 41

  Time to Take Charge | 44

3: Understanding Radiation Therapy | 46

  Members of the Radiation Oncology Team | 47

  Important Considerations | 50

  Side Effects of Radiation Therapy | 53

  Retreatment | 56

PART 2: How Do I Deal with This?

4: Lifestyle Management | 61

  Feel Empowered | 62

  Reduce Stress | 63

  Breathe Deeply | 65

  Consider Meditation | 65

  Move Your Muscles | 66

  Eat Well | 67

  Herbal and Dietary Supplements | 69

  Driving | 71

  Working | 74

  Support Groups | 75

  Cosmetic Issues | 76

  Creativity, Art, and Humor as Therapy | 78

5: Symptom Management and Palliative Care | 81

Symptoms | 82

"Big Picture" Topics to Keep in Mind | 90

6: Care of the Caregiver | 94

Presurgery | 95

During Treatment | 98

Recurrence | 109

7: Planning for Your Future: Managing Your Personal Affairs | 114

Murray Sagsveen, JD, and Laurie Hanson, JD

Your Emergency Notebook | 115

Informal and Formal Arrangements | 118

Durable Power of Attorney | 122

Trusts | 125

Health Care Directives|131

Guardianship and Conservatorship | 136

Your Will | 138

PART 3: What Can I and My Medical Team Do About It?

8: Benign Tumors | 143

Basics About Meningioma | 144

Treating Atypical and Malignant Meningiomas | 146

Pituitary Adenoma | 148

Acoustic Neuroma | 151

How Will Having One of These Tumors Affect My Life? | 152

9: Primary Brain Tumors | 154

   Understanding Your Treatment Options | 155

   Understanding Your Pathology Report | 161

   Radiation Therapy and Chemotherapy | 163

10: Metastatic Brain Tumors | 167

   Symptoms | 170

   Diagnosis | 171

   Treatment | 171

   Prognosis | 173

   Leptomeningeal Disease | 174

APPENDIX: GUIDE TO DRUGS PRESCRIBED FOR
   BRAIN TUMORS | 177
GLOSSARY | 182
ABOUT THE AUTHORS AND CONTRIBUTORS | 194
ABOUT THE AAN AND THE ABF | 197
INDEX | 199

ABOUT THE AAN'S *NEUROLOGY NOW*™ BOOK SERIES

Here is a question for you:

If you know more about your neurologic condition, will you do better than if you know less?

Well, it's not simply optimism but hard data that show that individuals who are more knowledgeable about their medical conditions *do have better outcomes*. So learning about your neurologic condition plays an important role in doing the very best you can. The main purpose of both the American Academy of Neurology's (AAN's) *Neurology Now*™ book series and *Neurology Now* magazine is to focus on the needs of people with neurologic disorders. Our goal is to view neurologic issues through the eyes of people with neurologic problems, in order to understand and respond to their practical day-to-day needs.

So, you are probably saying, *"Of course, knowledge is a good thing, but how can it change the course of my disease?"* Well, health care is really a two-way street. You need to find a knowledgeable and trusted neurologist; however, no physician can overcome the obstacle of working with inaccurate or incomplete information. Your physician is working to navigate the clues you provide in your own words combined with the clues from their neurologic examination, in order to arrive at an accurate diagnosis and respond to your individual needs. Many types of important clues exist, such as your description of your symptoms or your ability to identify how your neurologic condition affects your daily activities. Poor patient–physician communication inevitably results in less-than-ideal outcomes. This problem is well described by the old adage, "garbage in, garbage out." The better you pin down and communicate your main problem(s), the more likely you are to walk out of your doctor's office with the plan that is right for you. Your neurologist is the expert in your disorder, but you and your family are the experts in "you." Physician decision making is not a "one shoe fits all" enterprise, yet when accurate, individualized information is lacking, that's what it becomes.

Whether you are startled by hearing a new diagnosis or you come to this knowledge gradually, learning that you have a neurologic problem is jarring. Many neurologic disorders are chronic; you aren't simply adjusting to something new—you will need to deal with this disorder for the foreseeable future. In certain ways, life has changed. Now, there are two crucial "next steps": the first is finding good neurologic care for your problem, and the second is successfully adjusting to living with your condition. This second step depends on attaining knowledge of your condition, learning new skills to manage the condition, and finding the flexibility and resourcefulness to restore your quality of life. When successful, you regain your equilibrium and restore a sense of confidence and control that is the cornerstone of well-being.

When healthy adjustment does not occur following a new diagnosis, a sense of feeling out of control and overwhelmed often persists, and no doctor's prescription will adequately respond to this problem. Individuals who acquire good self-management skills are often able to recognize and understand new symptoms and take appropriate action. Conversely, those who are lacking in confidence may respond to the same symptom with a growing sense of anxiety and urgency. In the first case, "watchful waiting" or a call to the physician may result in resolution of the problem. In the second case, the uncertainty and anxiety often lead to multiple physician consultations, unnecessary new prescriptions, social withdrawal, or unwarranted hospitalization. Outcomes can be dramatically different depending on knowledge and preparedness.

Managing a neurologic disorder is new territory, and you should not be surprised that you need to be equipped with new information and a new skill set to effectively manage your condition. You will need to learn new words that describe both your symptoms and their treatment to communicate effectively with the members of your medical team. You will also need to learn how to gather accurate information about your condition when you need it and to avoid misinformation. Although all of your physicians document your progress in their medical records, keeping a personal journal about your neurologic condition will help you summarize and track all your medical information in one place. When you bring this journal with you as you go to see your physician, you will be able to provide more accurate information about your history and previous treatment. Your active and informed involvement in your care and decision making results in a better quality of care and better outcomes.

Your neurologic condition is likely to pose new challenges in daily activities, including interactions in your family, your workplace, and your social and recreational activities. How can you best manage your symptoms or your medication dosing schedule in the context of your normal activities? When should you disclose your diagnosis to others? *Neurology Now* Books provide you with the background you need, including the experiences of others who have faced similar problems, to guide you through this unfamiliar terrain. Our goal is to give you the resources you need to "take your doctor with you" when you confront these new challenges. We are committed to answering the questions and concerns of individuals living with neurologic disorders and their families in each volume of the *Neurology Now* book series. We want you to be as prepared and confident as possible to participate with your doctors in your medical care. Much care is taken to develop each book with you in mind. A special authorship model takes a multidisciplinary team approach to put together the most up-to-date, informative, and useful answers to the questions that most concern you—whether you find yourself in the unexpected role of patient or caregiver. Each authorship team includes neurologists with special expertise, along with a diversity of other contributors with special knowledge of the particular neurologic disorder. Depending on the specific condition, this includes rehabilitation specialists, nurses, social workers, and people or family members with important shared experiences. Professional writers work to ensure that we avoid "doctor talk," and easy-to-understand definitions of new terms appear on the page when a new word is introduced. Real-life experiences of patients and families are found throughout the text to illustrate important points. And feedback based on correspondence from *Neurology Now* magazine readers informs topics for new books and is integral to our quality improvement. These new features will be found in all books in the *Neurology Now* book series so that you can expect the same quality and patient-centered approach in every volume.

I hope that you have arrived at a new understanding of why "knowledge is empowering" when it comes to your medical care and that *Neurology Now* Books will serve as an important foundation for the new skills you need to be effective in managing a neurologic condition.

Lisa M. Shulman, MD
Editor-In-Chief, *Neurology Now* Book Series
and Professor of Neurology
University of Maryland School of Medicine

PREFACE

When I began my training as a neuro-oncologist, I was interested in helping patients with neurologic problems related to cancer survive longer and with a better quality of life. In the past 10 years, an explosion of knowledge has bettered both variables, and there is growing optimism for the ongoing development of improved treatments.

What I was not prepared for, however, was the profound impact the "illness narrative" of my patients would have on my own life. Listening to my patients and their caregivers share their experiences living with a life-threatening cancer diagnosis has been humbling, profoundly moving, but also at times surprisingly light hearted. For this reason my coauthors and I chose to focus less on treatment specifics, which can change, and more on the human aspects of relationships, emotions, and coping skills that will help you get through a serious illness. Our patients' stories are rich and full of wisdom; we hope you find them helpful.

Lynne P. Taylor, MD

ACKNOWLEDGMENTS

Lynne Taylor, MD
I would like to thank my sons, Ben and Chris, and my husband, Bruce Bagamery, PhD, for their constancy and gentle encouragement.

Alyx B. Porter Umphrey, MD
I'd like to thank my parents, my teachers (both formal and informal), my village of support, and most of all, Dr. Gregory Umphrey, Rylan, and Makena for lovingly supporting my numerous attempts at superhero status.

Diane Richard
I'd like to thank my husband, Todd Melby, for always lending me an ear; my co-authors, Lynne and Alyx, for their brilliance, tenacity, warmth, and humor; and Andrea Weiss at AAN, for giving me the opportunity.

Part 1

Where Do I Begin?

Introduction

The mind is its own place, and in itself can make a heaven of hell, a hell of heaven.

—John Milton, *Paradise Lost*

If you are reading this book, chances are high that either you or someone you care about has been diagnosed with a brain tumor. This particular diagnosis is one of the scariest imaginable and also one for which it is impossible to be prepared. Your doctor likely provided you with a lot of information, some of which you may remember now, some of which you may not. Yet, to face this challenge, you will want to be armed with as much information as possible. Many good resources exist, thankfully, and foremost among them is your medical team.

This book can serve as another resource. It is a comprehensive, physician-prepared guide to brain tumors—for those that originate in the brain, whether benign or malignant, and also for those that spread from elsewhere. It is designed to be medically authoritative, helpful, and, above all, valuable. You may find that it is a source you return to numerous times, whenever you have new questions, run across unfamiliar terminology, are looking to research treatment options, or could use a little inspiration from those who have been in your shoes.

"From the time he was diagnosed, it was clear we wouldn't say, 'We'll get around to that sometime,'" says Andy, younger brother of Richard, a landscape architect specializing in wetlands mitigation. Avid cyclists, the brothers have taken an almost-annual mountain bike trip throughout Richard's

17-year journey with recurrent oligodendroglioma tumors of the right temporal lobe. "It's definitely made it clear you have to live life," Andy says.

You've heard the diagnosis. You've clutched the hand of the loved one beside you. Now, to make the most of your medical care, there are some important next steps.

Step 1: Take a Deep Breath

Amid a raging flood of emotions, questions, worries, and information that may have little meaning to you, inhale once...twice...three times ... and remember this: You are not alone. Not only do you have the support of the people who know and love you, but you also are supported by the many physicians and health care professionals who have dedicated their careers to helping you through this moment and the many moments to come. This also holds true for caregivers, whose minds may be racing with concern, confusion, and what's next. No one expects you to feel or behave in any way other than how you are right now. The best things you can do are breathe and begin to gather up your reserves.

Step 2: Seek Out Information

This book is an ideal starting place because it provides critical information about types and possible causes of brain tumors, describes common symptoms, and defines the roles of your medical team. It also offers diagnostic criteria, addresses care and treatment options, empowers you to take charge of your legal and financial duties, and helps you marshal your internal and external strength to cope with an unquestionably challenging illness—whether it be through spiritual, intellectual, athletic, social, or creative means. It will also lead you to additional useful resources and support groups.

Additional Sources

Doctor's Office

Your medical team is a frontline resource for you now. During visits, ask your doctors or their staff for copies of all clinical notes, operative reports, test results, and films that have been done. Gathering such information is an important step to ensure that time spent with your medical team is efficient and that you have ready access for future reference. A copy of this information should be given to your treating physicians and another kept in your personal file.

Second Opinions

Because a brain tumor is a serious and potentially fatal diagnosis, it is wise to seek a second opinion. If you have an open relationship with your primary doctor, ask for his or her recommendations for this second opinion. Or use the Internet or other tool to research whether you live near a cancer center or neurologic clinic where you will most likely find an expert in the treatment and management of brain tumors, called a neuro-oncologist.

The Internet

In your quest for information, your first instinct may be to log on. Of course, the Internet is a wonderful tool that's always available—particularly during those 3:00 a.m. wakeups when your thoughts are bouncing off the bedposts—and can be a source of excellent information. But a word of caution is in order: be careful and also a bit skeptical about what you read because misinformation is rampant online. Choose credible sites for your research, and use that knowledge to supplement what you hear from your doctor. Websites of national foundations geared toward brain tumor research are typically a good place to start as are the websites of major reputable medical centers. Your doctor may also provide you with his or her preferred information sources online in order to help you focus your efforts. Early in the information-gathering stage, chat rooms tend to be less helpful and may be sources of misinformation.

Local Groups

Brain tumor support groups in your community are invaluable. Such groups can be places to develop new relationships for both patients and caregivers and to learn from the trials and triumphs of your peers. You may also hear about new clinical trials and medications that may be pertinent to your care or about helpful professionals in your area.

Step 3: Assemble Your Team

Many factors will play a role in your treatment, and your team of brain tumor specialists will no doubt reflect this complexity. Most teams consist of a neurologist or neuro-oncologist, a neurosurgeon, a radiation oncologist, and a medical oncologist. As a patient or caregiver, you may need to take an active role in assembling your medical team, or your neuro-oncologist may guide you. How these team members interact is discussed in depth in Chapter 2, "Diagnosing Your Brain Tumor."

Here's a quick description of your team's roles:

Neurologist: A doctor who specializes in diseases of the central and peripheral nervous system.

Neuro-oncologist: A neurologist who has received specialty training in cancers and tumors of the central and peripheral nervous systems, and who can treat both your neurologic symptoms as well as administer chemotherapy for treatment.

Neurosurgeon: A doctor who operates on the brain, spinal cord, and nerves.

Medical oncologist: An internal medicine doctor who has received special training in cancer and administers chemotherapies for treatment.

Radiation oncologist: A doctor who has received special training to administer radiation therapy to assist in the treatment of malignancies or cancers.

Step 4: Keep a Journal

Perhaps you've always kept a diary—or thought about doing so. This diagnosis offers an undeniable prompt to begin a journal or log to record symptoms, treatments, and discussions with doctors. If you are a caregiver, your assistance with this task is extremely helpful, as your loved one may at times feel overwhelmed. Although it will probably seem tedious at first, the value is well worth the effort. The practice of journaling can be empowering for both of you, and it also serves as a benchmark against which you can measure how much you have learned together. It will also be a relief to have this information readily accessible from one appointment to the next. Make sure to use it to record questions that come up between appointments, and bring it to every doctor's visit; that way, you will always have your thoughts at hand when the doctor asks, "Do you have any questions?" Because, beyond a doubt, you will.

Chapter 1

A Look Inside Your Brain

The brain is the most complex organ in the body; yet, despite many scientific advances, it remains the least understood and most mysterious. One thing is clear: Your brain is what makes you, you. It plays an essential role in shaping your personality, forming and keeping memories, managing your emotions, bringing balance and speed to your stride, and determining whether you are athletic, good at games like Pictionary, agile in foreign languages, remember jokes, prefer spicy or sweet flavors, and are able to sense the world's rich surroundings as you navigate your daily life.

In this chapter, you will learn the following:

- **How the brain is organized**
- **Why the location of a brain tumor matters**
- **How primary and secondary tumors differ**
- **How benign and malignant tumors differ**
- **What the basic tumor types are**
- **About the risk factors for getting a brain tumor**
- **Common symptoms of brain tumors**
- **Current technologies for reaching a diagnosis**

Basics About the Brain

The **central nervous system (CNS)** is composed of the brain and the spinal cord. The brain is housed within the skull and is protected by thin coverings or membranes, called the dura and the meninges. The brain is a spongy mass of nerve cells, fluids, and tissues that connects to the spinal cord (Figure 1–1).

Areas within the brain are identified a few different ways. The primary division is by its largest components, the two **cerebral hemispheres**, which are then divided into right and left. In most people, the left hemisphere is the dominant side, handling language and higher functions, such as strength and sensation in the right side of the body.

Each hemisphere is made up of four **lobes: frontal, parietal, temporal,** and **occipital.** The frontal lobes house our personality and make us who we are. Executive functioning, meaning the skills we have as human beings as distinct from other mammals—such as critical thinking and decision making—also comes from

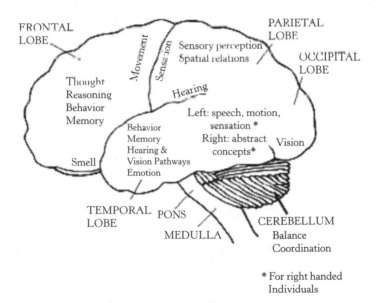

FRONTAL LOBE

PARIETAL LOBE

OCCIPITAL LOBE

Movement

Sensation

Sensory perception
Spatial relations

Thought
Reasoning
Behavior
Memory

Hearing

Left: speech, motion,
sensation *

Right: abstract
concepts*

Vision

Behavior
Memory
Hearing &
Vision Pathways
Emotion

Smell

TEMPORAL LOBE

PONS

MEDULLA

CEREBELLUM
Balance
Coordination

* For right handed
Individuals

FIGURE 1–1 A side view of the various lobes of the brain. Names of the lobes are in capital letters. Functions are listed in normal type.

this area. The parietal lobes help us to decipher direction and aid in visual-spatial orientation. The temporal lobes contain the main structures for thinking, memory, and language; they are also most prone to seizures. The occipital lobes help our eyes interpret what we see.

The **brainstem** is the stalk upon which the cerebral hemispheres sit. The brainstem is further divided into the **midbrain, pons,** and **medulla oblongata**. The midbrain, pons, and medulla oblongata supply basic matter for our cranial nerves and support vital functions such as breathing, heart rate, and wakefulness. The brainstem tapers down to form the spinal cord at the base of the skull, then travels through the spine to animate our limbs. Located in the back of the brain, the **cerebellum** is the balance center, helping us maintain posture and coordination.

There are **12 pairs of cranial nerves**, most of which originate in the brainstem; the first and second cranial nerves—olfactory and optic—are exceptions (Figure 1–2).

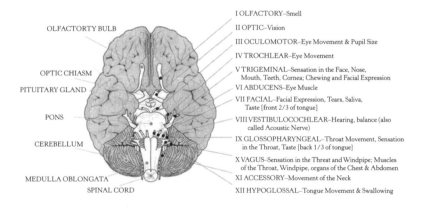

FIGURE 1–2 A view from underneath the brain showing the 12 cranial nerves and explaining their functions.

The **first cranial nerve (the olfactory nerves)** travels along the inferior, or underneath, portion of the frontal lobes and provides our sense of smell. With injury to the olfactory nerve, either from trauma in which it is stretched and broken or with compression from the swelling of a tumor, the senses of smell and taste can be damaged.

The second cranial nerve (the **optic nerves)** travels from the brain out to the eye itself and supports vision. It can be damaged by tumor growth on or near the nerve, causing diminished vision or visual loss on the affected side.

The third **(oculomotor)**, fourth **(trochlear)**, and sixth **(abducens)** cranial nerves originate in the midbrain and pontine portions of the brainstem and are vital for pupil and eye-muscle movements. With the impairment of any of these nerves, anywhere from the point of origin through its course as it exits the brain and stimulates the eye muscles, an individual may lose proper eye movement, causing **diplopia** (double vision).

The fifth cranial nerve **(trigeminal nerve)** originates within the pons and provides sensation to the face and strength to the muscles that help us chew.

The seventh cranial nerve **(facial nerve)** originates within the pons. It provides input to our facial muscles, allowing us to smile, grimace, wink, and make other nonverbal expressions, and, to a lesser extent, supports our sense of taste. It also controls some of the small muscles in the ear that regulate volume of sounds. Impairment of the facial nerve may cause facial paralysis (Bell's palsy) as well as diminished taste and heightened perception of sounds.

The eighth cranial nerve **(vestibulocochlear nerve)** originates in the pons and medulla and sends input for hearing and balance. Disturbance of the eighth cranial nerve can cause deafness and ringing in the ears on the affected side, along with vertigo (dizziness).

The following cranial nerves originate in the medulla oblongata:

The ninth cranial nerve (**glossopharyngeal nerve**) provides input for taste, salivation, and swallowing.

The tenth cranial nerve (**vagus nerve**) mediates swallowing and speech and stimulates some of our abdominal organs. It is the longest cranial nerve, and interruptions in its pathway can cause hoarseness, **dysphagia** (impaired swallowing), and **dysarthria** (slurred speech).

The eleventh cranial nerve (**accessory nerve**) stimulates the muscles that control head and neck movement.

The twelfth cranial nerve (**hypoglossal nerve**) provides input for tongue movement.

The **pituitary gland** lies within the skull and is connected to, although is technically outside of, the brain. It produces and regulates hormones to keep our body in balance. Such hormones are important for physical growth, sexual function, and regulating levels of salt and adrenaline in the body. Therefore, if a tumor grows within or compresses the pituitary gland, a hormone imbalance may occur. Furthermore, because of the pituitary gland's closeness to the optic nerves, loss of vision is possible.

As you can see, the brain is a very complicated organ. Because of its complexity, the development of a brain tumor may be accompanied by a variety of symptoms, depending on the location and type. The increased mass can raise the pressure within the skull, resulting in symptoms such as headaches, nausea, vomiting, sleepiness, or even loss of consciousness.

As tempting as it may be, be careful not to draw conclusions based on one specific symptom. For instance, a disruption in the vision system may indicate a problem in any of a number of locations, from the eye itself, to the optic nerve, the deep internal structures within the brain and brainstem, the temporal lobe, or the occipital lobe. The job of the medical team is to determine where in the pathway the problem lies and to order the appropriate testing to confirm a diagnosis.

Understanding Brain Tumors

A brain tumor, like other types of tumors, is an abnormal collection of cells that multiply and may cause damage to the surrounding tissue and involved organs. Brain cancer makes up only 1.4 percent of all cancer cases. Nonetheless, it is one of the most difficult types of cancer to fight.

One reason for this challenge is the vast variety of tumor types; there are more than 120 different types of brain tumors.

Brain tumors are classified as either **primary** or **secondary**. A primary brain tumor means the cancerous cells originate in the brain. A secondary—or **metastatic**—brain tumor is a mass of cells that originates elsewhere in the body, then spreads through the bloodstream to the brain in a process known as metastasis. The most common secondary brain tumors arise from the lung, breast, kidney, colon, and blood cells (lymphoma).

Once a diagnosis is made, the medical team will also attempt to determine whether the tumor is **intra-axial** (within the central nervous system) or **extra-axial** (located outside the central nervous system). Years ago, such a determination was difficult to make. Today, through technological advances in neuroimaging, medical experts now have more accurate information from which to reach a decision. This classification provides clues about the tumor type and will inform the future treatment options and plan.

What makes brain tumors unique among all types of cancer is that they occur in the skull. The skull is an ideal container for brain, blood, and spinal fluid. Nevertheless, it is a fixed space that allows precious little room for anything else to reside within it. As a result, a tumor's cellular mass takes up room within that bony box, invading healthy tissue, damaging nearby neurological pathways, and building pressure on sensitive areas of the brain that are essential to an individual's cognitive, physical, and sensory functions. Most types of primary brain tumors are similar in that they tend to share characteristics, such as their shape, the way they spread, their location, and their related symptoms. Understanding these characteristics aids your doctor in arriving at a diagnosis and charting a course to manage the brain tumor.

Location, Location, Location

Like that old real estate saying goes, it's all about location, location, location. When it comes to understanding brain tumors, much is determined by location as well. Because of the complex duties handled by specific areas of the brain and the intricate web of nerves that make those duties possible, the location of the tumor gives important clues to the cause (known in clinical terms as "etiology") and the best approach to managing the tumor. The location of the tumor will determine whether there are dramatic symptoms or none at all (Figure 1–1).

Some symptoms are indeed subtle, as Paul observed. On two successive days, Paul found himself typing gobbledygook on the keyboard, his right hand divorced from his left. "I looked down at the gibberish and thought, 'This is wrong.'" Paul's peripheral vision had been impaired by a tumor called a **glioblastoma multiforme** located in the left occipital lobe. Looking back, Paul says, with a touch of irony, that the tumor probably also accounted for the sudden occurrence of wild swings on the fairway.

Brain tumors are classified as either benign or malignant, although this classification is not always precise.

Benign tumors tend to grow slowly and may not be associated with any symptoms for a long time. They are most likely to be detected incidentally, or by accident. In many cases, an imaging study is done of the brain for some other reason, such as after a car accident or a fall. Only at that time is the tumor detected. A benign tumor is less likely to cause damage to surrounding tissue or organs, typically does not recur, and rarely leads to death.

Malignant tumors tend to grow aggressively and may spread to surrounding tissues by direct invasion or through the bloodstream. Despite adequate treatment, they may recur either in the same place or a distant location, for instance, traveling from the breast or lung to the brain (See Chapter 10). In contrast, primary tumors that arise in the brain rarely spread beyond the brain. A malignant tumor, if left untreated, will ultimately lead to death.

The symptoms and treatment approaches of brain tumors vary widely depending on their location in the brain, whether the tumor is primary or secondary, benign or malignant, and many other factors. Your treatment will be specifically tailored for you, based on the tumor's characteristics (as seen through sophisticated imaging technology), your symptoms, and the tumor type, as well as your general medical health and the possible side effects of potential treatments.

Common Primary Brain Tumors

Each year, according to the National Brain Tumor Society, approximately 190,000 Americans are diagnosed with primary or metastatic (secondary) brain tumors. Primary brain tumors are known by the type of brain cell it originated from. For example, an astrocytoma develops from an astrocyte, and an oligodendro-glioma arises from an oligodendrocyte. The type of tumor you have and where it occurs will govern everything from your symptoms, to your medical treatment, and to your prognosis and likelihood of recovery (Figure 1–3 to Figure 1–5).

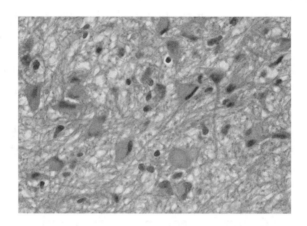

FIGURE 1-3 Astrocytoma.

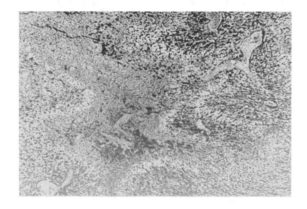

FIGURE 1-4 Glioblastoma multiforme (GBM).

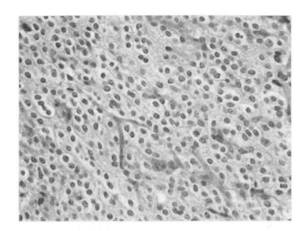

FIGURE 1-5 Oligodendroglioma.

Astrocytoma and Glioma

Astrocytoma and glioma are the most common forms of primary brain tumor, named for their cells of origin, the star-shaped glial cell (astrocyte). When functioning properly, the astrocyte provides structural as well as nutritional support for the neuron, or nerve cell. Astrocytomas tend to occur in adults but may also occur in children. Based on the way the tissue looks under the microscope, a pathologist will grade the astrocytoma in four stages, 1 to 4, from least to most aggressive. A grade 3 astrocytoma is also called an **anaplastic astrocytoma**. A grade 4 astrocytoma is called a **glioblastoma multiforme (GBM)**. A GBM is the most invasive form of glial tumor and grows rapidly.

Characteristics

Grade 3 and 4 astrocytomas are also known as high-grade gliomas. When looked at through sophisticated imaging technology, they appear to have many tendrils and are highly visible with contrast dye. The area around the tumor may also be swollen or shifted.

Common Symptoms
High-grade gliomas tend to grow aggressively and may cause neurologic symptoms in a rapid or sudden manner, often in just days or weeks.

Oligodendroglioma

The second most common primary brain tumor, oligodendrogliomas arise from oligodendrocytes, which are cells within the brain that make myelin. Myelin is a fatty substance that covers and "insulates" the neurons, helping to transmit impulses between neurons. Oligodendrogliomas are an important subset of brain tumor because they are much more sensitive to chemotherapy than astrocytomas. Therefore, carefully noting the presence of the oligodendroglial cells is an important job for the neuropathologist and will be explained further in Chapter 8.

Characteristics
Typically slow growing, oligodendrogliomas may look calcified on imaging studies.

Common Symptoms
Slow, progressive neurologic dysfunction and seizures.

Ependymoma

An ependymoma is a tumor that comes from the ependymal cells, which line the fluid-filled spaces in the brain. A less common type of tumor, ependymomas tend to form within the brain or spinal cord, and they may metastasize from the brain to the spine.

Characteristics
Commonly found in the brain in children and in the spine in adults.

Common Symptoms
Headaches, signs of increased intracranial pressure (a constellation of headache, blurred vision, nausea, and vomiting) or trouble with walking and balance.

Pituitary Tumor

The pituitary gland is located right above the nerves that support vision. Therefore, a growing pituitary mass may cause visual problems.

Characteristics
Most pituitary tumors are benign and occur in adults. They are often slow growing and the tumor itself may secrete hormones.

Common Symptoms
Abnormal hormone levels, headaches, and changes in vision.

Meningioma

Accounting for about 20 percent of brain tumors among adults, meningiomas arise from the cells that cover the brain and spine, called meninges. Among the most common incidentally diagnosed tumors, meningiomas tend to be benign, although once removed they can recur.

Characteristics
Meningiomas are usually slow growing and are more common in women.

Common Symptoms
The symptoms caused by meningiomas vary based on location. Many patients have no symptoms at all and the tumor is found by accident. Some patients may experience headache, seizures, or weakness or numbness of the face or limbs.

A Search for Why

Why me? Is it because I use my cell phone a lot? Or because I heat my food with a microwave? Or live near a power line, or radio tower? Eat too much junk food? Not enough flax, kale, or broccoli? Or did I somehow inherit it?

Such questions are common among those recently diagnosed with a brain tumor. It's tempting to wonder whether or to what extent our environment, our activity, our diet, or our disposition has contributed to our state of health. Research has proved vexingly inconclusive about the causes of and possible risks for developing brain tumors.

> Jenny is like most people with brain tumors—baffled as to why she developed not one, but two, glioblastoma multiforme tumors over 12 years. A lover of nature, fresh air, healthy foods, meaningful work, and meditation, she still asks herself, "Why me? I'm very hearty. I eat vegetables."

Known and Possible Causes

Assigning risk factors for brain tumors is controversial, and not much concrete evidence exists. Prior exposure to brain radiation is the most solid risk factor for devloping a primary brain tumor. Historically, studies have shown an increased incidence of primary tumors among atomic bomb survivors, such as for residents of Nagasaki and Hiroshima, Japan. In the development of childhood brain tumors, the significance of prenatal exposure to radiation is

TABLE 1-1 Rare Genetic Syndromes Associated with Heightened Risk of Tumor Development

Syndrome Name	Tumor Types
Neurofibromatosis 2 (NF-2)	Acoustic neuromas, astrocytomas, and meningiomas
Hereditary non-polyposis colon cancer (HNPCC) or Lynch syndrome	Increased incidence of colon cancer and brain tumors in members of the same family
Li-Fraumeni	Sarcomas, breast cancer, and brain cancer
Von Hippel-Lindau	Tumors of the brain, spinal cord, kidney, and adrenal gland

unclear. There's also limited evidence linking X-ray exposure during dental procedures to an increased risk of brain tumors. It is also debatable whether exposure to electromagnetic fields raises the risk of developing brain tumors in people who live near power plants. Most studies have shown no correlation, and the same is true for studies of cell phones and microwave ovens; none reliably demonstrates an increased risk, but studies are ongoing.

Possible dietary associations to cancer have also been the subject of abundant research. For instance, certain nitrate compounds present in meat have been linked by scientific study to an increased risk of brain tumors in animals; however, no such link has been shown in research in humans. Likewise, certain viruses and chemicals have been shown to cause brain tumors in animals; nevertheless, similar studies have proved inconclusive in humans. Smoking does not appear to increase the risk of primary brain tumors, although it certainly heightens the risk of lung cancer. No solid evidence exists to link certain professions associated with chemical exposures, or viral vaccinations or prescription medications, to the development of primary brain tumors.

Research into hereditary factors has linked certain rare genetic syndromes with an increased risk of brain tumor development. Make sure to inform your medical care team if your family history includes any of these syndromes (see Table 1–1).

Getting a Diagnosis

For about 2 years, Christopher had noticed things weren't quite right. He had headaches and his short-term memory "was shot."

"I became a creature of habit," he says. "I had to drive from point A to point B, or I'd get lost. I knew something was going on."

Then, a "headache from hell" set in—for 3 days. Christopher went to the emergency department, where a doctor "looked into my eyes very carefully, ordered a CT [computerized tomography] scan, and within an hour I was rushed to the surgeon," he says. The CT scan came back positive; there was a mass.

"Next thing I know there was a surgeon staring me in the face, telling me he had to cut a tumor out of my brain." The diagnosis, a low-grade oligodendroglioma in the right temporal lobe, "answered a lot of questions," he says. "My first thought was, it makes sense. My god, it makes sense." Having an explanation was important to Christopher. "No one wants to hear they have cancer," he says. "But I thought I was going crazy, that I was losing my mind. So in a way it was a relief. Now it's a matter of getting my life back."

Several steps typically occur before someone is given a brain tumor diagnosis. In most cases, an individual will seek treatment from his or her primary care doctor for various hard-to-explain symptoms. Such symptoms can include seizures, weakness or numbness on one side of the body, difficulty with balance or walking, trouble with speech or swallowing, and headaches.

Sometimes the symptoms are obvious; but others may be subtle, such as a change in personality or behavior. Many things can account for these subtle symptoms, such as stress or the need for a stronger eyeglass prescription, so alarm should not be your first reaction. Nevertheless, they may indicate something of concern taking place within the brain that could warrant further attention. Any symptom that's new, different, or worsening should prompt a call to the medical team.

Depending on the outcome of the visit, your doctor may refer you to a specialist, such as a neurologist—a medical doctor who specializes in diseases affecting the nervous system. At this point, the neurologist will gather a thorough clinical history, chronicling details about your symptoms and their progression. Next, the neurologist will perform a careful neurological examination, focusing on thinking and memory, language, strength, coordination, balance, sensation, and reflexes. The examination will also include a neuroimaging scan of your brain. Based on the results, the neurologist will then offer you his or her impressions and any recommendations for further testing, discussed in Chapter 2. Such testing may come quickly, should the neurologist detect a mass.

Chapter 2

Diagnosis

From his hotel room in India, pilot Jim was chatting over a Web cam with his wife, Sharolyn, when something suddenly went wrong. He couldn't put his thoughts together, she remembers, and his words came out ajumble. "I thought he was having a stroke," she says. Then he fell over the back of his chair. "I called the hotel and told them I wanted a doctor to go to his room," she says.

A brain tumor was discovered shortly thereafter at an Indian hospital. That was in May 2008. A week later, Jim was home, diagnosed with having a grade 4 astrocytoma, also known as a glioblastoma multiforme. Less than 3 weeks upon its discovery, the tumor was surgically removed, followed by radiation and chemotherapy.

Had Sharolyn not been face to face over Skype with Jim, or able to secure immediate medical attention, who can say what might have happened? Despite the thousands of miles that separated the couple, her quick action and the chain of events that followed played key roles in the diagnosis and treatment of Jim's brain tumor.

Diagnosing a brain tumor is a bit like solving a puzzle, only the stakes are significantly higher. By now, the doctor who detected your tumor is likely to have a general idea about its site, based on symptoms you have described. Now, the goal is to gather the specifics—because treating a brain tumor is all about precision. Early detection and timely treatment improve the likelihood of a positive outcome, so an accurate diagnosis is critical.

In this chapter, you will learn the following:

- **The common tests used to help achieve a diagnosis**
- **The roles of each member of your medical care team**
- **How to request a second opinion**
- **Where to find additional resources**
- **The role of a tumor board**
- **Ways to think about prognosis**
- **Suggestions for taking charge of your care**

Assessment and Plan

After you've given your health history and you've had a general medical and neurological examination, your neurologist will form an assessment and plan in which the most likely and most treatable diagnoses are considered first. The tests mentioned next are used to confirm a diagnosis and—ultimately—determine whether a **biopsy**, the surgical retrieval of a small portion of tumor tissue, or surgery will be useful in making a final diagnosis.

The first step involves imaging using either **computerized axial tomography (CT or "CAT") scan** (Figure 2–1) or **magnetic resonance imaging (MRI)** (Figure 2–2) technologies, or possibly both.

The patterns of abnormality found through these sophisticated imaging techniques provide useful clues regarding whether the tumor is malignant or benign, has arisen from within or outside of the brain, and if it appears to have originated in or traveled to the brain from elsewhere in the body. Scans that reveal multiple tumors spread throughout several lobes of the brain, in particular, raise the possibility of a brain **metastasis**.

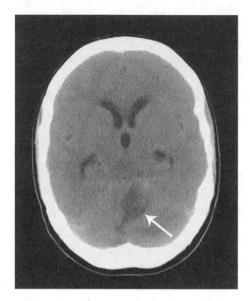

FIGURE 2-1 A computerized tomography (CT) image of the brain showing swelling in the left cerebellum and hydrocephalus (enlargement and obstruction of the lateral ventricles).

Despite the advances of modern neuroimaging, a solid diagnosis often requires further workup and testing. That's where the expertise of a **neuro-oncologist** comes in. Your brain tumor specialist will recommend further testing to help pinpoint a diagnosis. At the same time, he or she will attempt to rule out medical conditions that sometimes mimic brain tumors, such as brain infections or abscesses, strokes, benign calcifications, and, in rare cases, inflammatory or autoimmune disorders, such as multiple sclerosis.

Imaging Techniques

Computerized axial tomography (CT or "CAT") scan is a type of X-ray that provides information about the brain and skull. The procedure typically lasts 10 minutes while you lie on a moveable

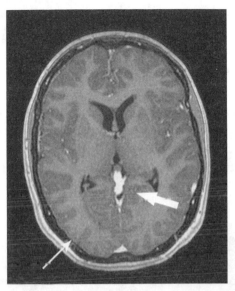

FIGURE 2-2 A magnetic resonance imaging (MRI) of the brain at the same level as the computerized tomography (CT) scan. Note the inferior evaluation of bone which was white on the CT image, but the superior detail of the anatomy of the brain, particularly vessels (thick arrow) and the cortical ribbon (thin arrow).

table that glides smoothly into the center of a doughnut-shaped machine. A **radiologist** may inject contrast dye, which highlights abnormal tissue, through an arm vein to render the tumor more visible. If you develop a rash or itching after the dye is administered, you must quickly alert someone, as it may be an allergic reaction. This reaction is common for people with known allergies to shellfish, which can contain iodine, the element used for CT contrast.

Magnetic resonance imaging (MRI) uses magnetic fields to take highly detailed three-dimensional images of the brain. For your safety, you will be asked to remove all clothes with metal parts and jewelry because of the magnets used in the technology. Expect to lie within the MRI cylinder for about 20 minutes to1 hour. Some people report feeling claustrophobic. If you expect this might be the case for you, let the staff know beforehand. You may be given a mild sedative to help you relax or referred to a center with an "open" MRI. However, a closed MRI is preferable as the images that result are of higher resolution and better quality. Again, a contrasting agent (unrelated to iodine) may be administered to help provide more detailed information about the tumor and the surrounding structures (Figure 2–3A to Figure 2–3C, Figure 2–4).

Your doctor may also order **X-rays** of your skull to determine whether the bone has changed its shape. This view could provide valuable information regarding the tumor's origin as well as its behavior.

An **angiogram** may be used to assess the blood vessels in the brain and, specifically, to study the blood supply to the tumor itself. A neuroradiologist (a doctor who specializes in interpreting

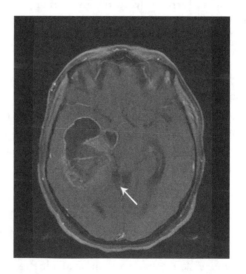

FIGURE 2–3A-C Three ways a glioblastoma can appear on a magnetic resonance imaging (MRI) scan.

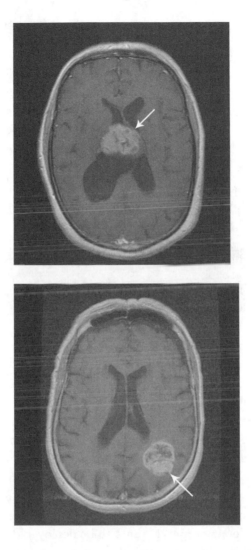

FIGURE 2-3A-C *Continued.*

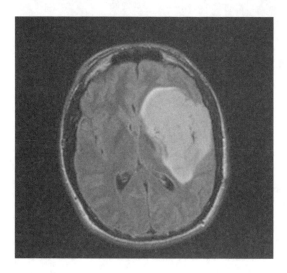

FIGURE 2-4 Typical magnetic resonance imaging appearance of an oligodedroglioma.

imaging studies of the brain) or a **neurosurgeon** commonly performs this procedure. It begins with the insertion of a catheter—a thin, flexible, plastic tube—into a blood vessel in the groin. It is then threaded up to the vessels that supply the brain. Next, contrast dye is injected to give the neuroradiologist a clearer view of the anatomy. This type of invasive angiogram makes it possible for the operator to watch the rate and direction of blood flow inside the artery in real time, showing how the blood is moving around a narrowed blood vessel. It also helps prepare for the use of small balloons or metal stents to be deployed during the procedure to treat the narrowed blood vessel. For tumor patients, the angiogram is often performed to find out about blood supply to the tumor. In this case, glue or other particles can be injected directly into tumor vessels to minimize the likelihood of tumor bleeding at a later surgery. Another option is a **magnetic resonance angiogram (MRA)**, a less invasive form of angiogram.

An MRA is performed much like an MRI, though it requires no needlestick to the groin area and takes just a few minutes longer. With an MRA, blood vessels are viewed without the dynamic information given by a standard angiogram about blood flow and with no opportunity to treat narrowed normal blood vessels or abnormal tumor vessels.

Several other imaging studies may be helpful for your doctors, including **magnetic resonance spectroscopy (MRS), positron emission tomography (PET)**, and **single-photon emission-computed tomography (SPECT)**. These studies provide information about blood flow to particular parts of the brain, as well as chemical characteristics of the tumors. Such studies are less common, available mostly at major medical centers across the country.

Your doctor may also order an **electroencephalogram (EEG)**. This electrophysiologic study provides information regarding the brain's tendency toward seizure, an interruption in normal brain functioning. Electrodes are glued to the scalp to make a brain wave recording. The procedure is painless and lasts about 30 to 45 minutes. Your doctor may request that you come to the appointment sleep deprived so that you can fall asleep during the test. The sleeping brain can provide a lot of valuable information.

Thus far, none of the testing should be painful for you—although the thought of all those tests may be unnerving. Being prepped for the contrast agent, commonly used in an MRI or CT scan, is possibly the most uncomfortable part; it requires a needle insertion, which connects to an intravenous (IV) tube through which the substance flows. Many report that the sensation is similar to donating blood.

The most invasive diagnostic procedure is, of course, surgical—either through biopsy or **gross total resection**, the removal of an entire tumor. Performed by a neurosurgeon, a biopsy involves drilling a small hole in the skull to obtain a sample of the tumor. During the procedure, some patients remain awake, while others are put under anesthesia. This is generally performed with IV medications while you are inside the MRI machine. Though you are awake, medications are used so that you will not remember the procedure. Depending on where the tumor is located, the surgeon may choose to remove the entire tumor or only a portion of it. Called a craniotomy, this surgery, which takes place in an operating room, involves the removal of a large plate of skull bone to create an opening through which to remove the tumor. After the surgery, the bone is replaced. The resulting scar is usually hidden within the hairline but will be visible until the scar heals. The tumor, or tumor sample, will then be given to a pathologist to examine under the microscope.

Supplemental Testing
Magnetic Resonance Spectroscopy (MRS)

Performed much like a brain MRI scan, MRS requires you to lie on a bed, which is inserted into a machine shaped like a tube. The machine's sensitive sensors allow the radiologist to place a small box or marker over a region of interest in the scan to measure the chemical content of the tissue. Its results can either confirm or deny the presence of cancerous tissue (Figure 2–5A and Figure 2–5B).

Positron Emission Tomography (PET)

This test can confirm the presence of cancerous tissue throughout the body and brain. It is most often used when the brain tumor is suspected to be metastatic, or having originated outside the brain. A radioactive sugar tracer is injected into a vein and given time to spread throughout the body (about 1 hour). (SPECT, a procedure similar to PET, uses thallium instead of radioactive sugar for a tracer.) A three-dimensional whole-body image

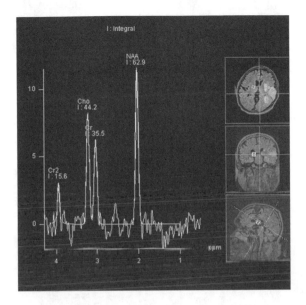

FIGURE 2-5A Magnetic resonance spectroscopy (MRS) is a technique that shows the chemical content of the area in question. Note the peaks of NAA, creatinine, and choline that are routinely sampled. This voxel (little box) is placed over normal brain.

follows. The image reveals areas where the radioactive tracer has been absorbed, a clue to a possible cancer. Detection of abnormal tissue in a lymph node, the lung, the breast, or in another organ is helpful in that it might avert the need for a biopsy of brain tissue. A biopsy of bodily tissue is relatively less complicated than that of the brain, which is a much more invasive procedure.

Lumbar Puncture

Also called a **spinal tap,** this test involves the insertion of a small needle into the spinal fluid space between the backbones (similar to an epidural procedure used to ease the pain of childbirth). The spinal fluid is then analyzed under the microscope for abnormal

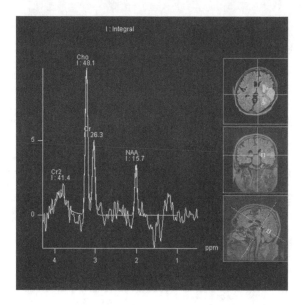

FIGURE 2-5B Voxel (little box) is placed over the tumor showing that the NAA peak has dropped below the choline and creatinine peaks. NAA is present in normal brain cells. Choline and creatinine are metabolic by-products of cell growth, so therefore suggest these areas are likely representative of a tumor.

cells, sugars, and certain proteins seen in people with multiple sclerosis. Special testing for viruses and bacteria is also commonly performed.

Blood Tests

Certain types of tumors secrete "tumor markers" that can be measured in the blood. These markers often indicate the location of an underlying tumor, such as of the lung or breast. Various blood tests are helpful in yielding a diagnosis. For instance, an abnormal complete blood count can suggest an underlying viral or bacterial infection. Serum protein electrophoresis, when combined with an analysis of spinal fluid, may reveal markers for multiple sclerosis. Testing for human immunodeficiency virus (HIV) is sometimes performed to detect risk for the development of certain brain tumors. Also, people suspected of having tumors of the pituitary gland are likely to have their hormone levels checked through blood tests.

Bone Marrow Biopsy

This test is helpful in detecting leukemia and lymphoma, cancers of the blood or bone marrow. It involves sampling bone marrow in the pelvis by needle.

Visual Field Examination

This test is performed while the individual is seated either with his or her head inside a computer field or facing a large black screen. It involves the projection of items of differing size and brightness, with the goal of mapping out the central and peripheral field of vision of each eye. Such information can be helpful in determining how much tissue can be removed for tumors affecting vision.

Getting the Medical Help You Need

The discovery of a brain tumor tends to occur abruptly and unexpectedly. It's possible your symptoms sent you straight to your local hospital's emergency department, or your family or internal medicine doctor suspected a problem, which was later confirmed by an MRI brain scan. Either way, chances are good your next visit was to a neurosurgeon. This step is certainly appropriate. Nonetheless, you might wish to consider getting a second opinion or an evaluation by a neurologist or a neuro-oncologist. Though time is of the essence for the treatment of many tumors, another qualified confirmation of your initial diagnosis and treatment approach is imperative, particularly if surgery has been recommended.

How to Seek a Second Opinion

The first step is to inform your doctor of your intentions and to request his or her recommendations. A second opinion from someone whose expertise is valued by your doctor is ideal. If you feel uncomfortable making this request, or if you feel that it is unwelcome, you may want to reach out beyond your immediate medical community.

Specialty medical societies are also good sources for referrals. The Society for Neuro-Oncology lists members who are brain tumor specialists on its Web site (http://www.soc-neuro-onc.org). The National Cancer Institute posts listings of cancer clinical trials (http://www.clinicaltrials.gov). These institutions and their Web sites are good sources of accurate information. Also, national patient advocacy groups such as the National Brain Tumor Society (http://www.braintumor.org) and the American Brain Tumor Association (http://www.abta.org) have knowledgeable staffs that can help answer your questions.

Other possibilities include the following:

Tumor boards: Most large medical centers dedicated to the care of people with brain tumors host multidisciplinary tumor boards. These groups of specialists meet regularly to review specific patients diagnosed with brain tumors. They review clinical histories, X-rays,

(Continued)

(Continued)

and **pathology** reports and discuss the best treatment. At the conclusion, a joint recommendation is made and communicated to the patient, who can choose to follow or reject it. Although these boards are helpful in reaching the best group decision regarding patient care, they are no substitute for the one-on-one relationship between patient and doctor.

Virtual tumor boards: An emerging trend, it is now possible to find a virtual tumor board at some of the larger medical centers via the Internet. Either patient or doctor can send the clinical history and all of the important MRI scans to request a "virtual" second opinion. A fee is typically required and, because the individual cannot be examined, the true value of such second opinions is unclear. If you desire a second opinion of the highest quality, it is best to travel to another medical center. Once there, you can give your medical history, have a physical and neurologic examination, and have your MRI scans reviewed in person.

Assembling Your Team

Ultimately, it is your choice who is on your medical team. Because a brain tumor is a complex diagnosis, you will be working with doctors who manage seizure disorders, evaluate your neurologic tests, read your MRI scans, and perform any necessary surgery. Until now, your daily life may not have included many of these professionals. Now, you will need to seek them out, helped by your primary care doctor or neurologist. Ideally, members of your medical care team will not only excel at doing their jobs, but they will also be good at responding to your questions and concerns and explaining the choices you have. What's more, they should be willing to teach you how to read your tests and scans and to monitor your symptoms. The size and nature of your community, the availability of medical experts, and other factors will, of course, play a role in your choices. Also, if possible:

- Locate a neuro-oncologist to anchor your team. Typically a neurologist with additional training in oncology or cancer treatment, a neuro-oncologist is specially trained to care for people with brain tumors. However, some neuro-oncologists are **medical oncologists** or neurosurgeons with additional training. Such experiences can shape a neuro-oncologist's approach to treatment and the relative strengths he or she brings to your team.
- Choose a board-certified doctor for your care team. You can always ask your doctor for confirmation of board certification, or you can often find this information online.

Other members of your care team:

- **Clinical trial staff**: Trained specifically as clinical trial coordinators, these individuals are expected to know the minute details of a particular clinical trial, to coordinate care with your medical care team, and to ensure the ethical conduct of the trial.
- **Medical oncologist**: An internal medicine expert specifically trained to administer chemotherapy treatment. During treatment cycles, chemotherapy drugs are taken by mouth or injected into a vein. These treatment cycles can last several hours a day every 2, 6, or 8 weeks, depending on the type of chemotherapy used. Medical oncologists are skilled at interpreting bloodwork, ensuring that chemotherapy patients are treated safely and effectively. They generally are not trained

to perform neurologic examinations or to interpret brain scans.

- **Neurorehabilitation**: This term describes a wide range of rehabilitation providers—speech therapists, physical therapists, occupational therapists, neuropsychologists, physiatrists (a doctor specializing in physical medicine and rehabilitation)—dedicated to your rehabilitation and return to optimal neurologic functioning.
- Neurosurgeon: Often the first doctor you will see, a neurosurgeon gathers your medical history, evaluates your initial examination, reviews your brain scans, and, if needed, determines the appropriate surgical intervention. So important for the initial diagnosis, the neurosurgeon will often not remain an active member of your care team, but she or he may return if another surgical procedure is needed.
- Pathologist/**Neuropathologist**: A doctor who evaluates tumor tissue on a glass slide through a microscope, and also the reaction of those cells to special chemical markers. This doctor helps your neurosurgeon to evaluate your tumor during surgery. The tissue is "flash-frozen" and a "frozen section" diagnosis is made to help your surgeon plan the extent of the operation. Afterward, a special fixing technique is used to preserve the tissue for evaluation several days later, leading to a final diagnosis. Once the slides are made and the tissue blocks are cut, these materials can be sent to other pathologists at other institutions, if necessary, for a second opinion.
- **Radiation oncologist**: A doctor who applies radiation therapy to brain tumors. These invisible radiation beams are directed at the tumor's location while you are lying on the treatment couch. First, the radiation oncologist takes a medical history, performs a physical examination, and reviews your pathology and MRI scans. The plan for radiation treatment will be informed by your MRI scans and made with the

behind-the-scenes help of a medical physicist. The radiation oncologist monitors your health and well-being weekly over the course of your radiation treatment, but then his or her active participation diminishes once radiation therapy is completed, typically in 3 to 6 weeks.

- **Radiation technician**: Your daily contact during radiation therapy, the radiation technician sees to the technical details of your radiation therapy, manages the machine, and supervises quality control.
- Radiologist/**Neuroradiologist**: These doctors read and interpret your CT and MRI scans. They are either radiologists trained to read X-rays and scans of every kind, or specialists in neuroradiology trained specifically to read radiographic studies of the nervous system. Most radiologists read scans performed at a specific institution and will compare your MRI scans to your prior studies. If your treatment period is long, or if you move from place to place during its course, make sure that you have another doctor (likely a neurologist or neuro-oncologist) who can help you review your films over time, not just compared to your last study. Indeed, request that your scans be placed on a compact disk so you have a personal copy to use for backup documentation.
- Registered nurses (RNs) and advanced registered nurse practitioners (ARNPs): Registered nurses and nurse practitioners work with your doctors to ensure you receive the very best care. Nurses help administer chemotherapy, talk to you about side effects, help you manage your symptoms, and educate you about the tumor type, treatment, and what to expect during your care.
- Social worker: A specially trained expert on finances, insurance options, and family communication and resources who can also help with counseling and psychosocial support.

Finalizing Your Treatment Team

Although many of the providers listed in this chapter will actively participate in your care team, you may not meet all of them. Some, however, will start to feel like family; indeed, many people with brain tumors and their caregivers report enjoying long-standing relationships with their care providers, years beyond the end of their treatment. Others you'll know for a brief, intense time. For instance, your neurosurgeon and radiation therapist will perform their roles expertly, then move on to the treatment of others.

Your task now is to decide how you want your health and well-being to be followed and by whom. You will need a single doctor—either a neurologist or neuro-oncologist—who can treat most of your concerns and also evaluate your neurologic tests and brain scans with you over time. If your community lacks neuro-oncologists, a neurologist paired with a medical oncologist might make a good team. The medical oncologist can manage your chemotherapy, if needed, and a general neurologist can evaluate your neurologic examination and your brain MRI scans. Sometimes, doctors in your local community can work with neuro-oncologists elsewhere. That way your day-to-day care occurs at home, where you are surrounded by your support system, and you can travel to your neuro-oncologist at 3- to 6-month intervals to have your MRI scan performed. Another possibility is for your local doctors to manage your care, having them send you to the neuro-oncologist only if some unexpected neurologic problem should occur.

Understanding Your Prognosis

Upon a diagnosis of a brain tumor or metastasis, it's human nature to wonder what the future might hold. Contemporary medical literature has many more articles devoted to diagnosis and treatment than to prognosis—yet this topic is the single one most people hope to find an answer to. As you prepare to ask your doctors about your prognosis, it may help to consider the most important prognostic indicators, or pieces of information known to affect outcome.

Important Prognostic Indicators for Primary Brain Tumors

A. Good prognostic indicators
1. Age at diagnosis: Younger than 60 years is associated with better outcomes
2. Extent of tumor removal, particularly if removal of all visible tumor has occurred
3. Normal neurologic examination after surgery
4. High performance status (i.e., no symptoms and able to carry on with all the usual activities of daily living without help)

B. Variable prognostic indicators
1. Pathology: Each tumor type will have its own associated prognosis

Important Prognostic Indicators for Secondary (Metastatic) Brain Tumors

A. Limited disease in the rest of the body
B. Small numbers of metastatic tumors
C. Small size of metastatic tumors

Statistics for survival can be presented in many different, and often confusing, ways. The percentage of people alive at 1, 5, and 10 years after a diagnosis may be a medical fact, but it does little to help you know what to expect for yourself. Also, statistics do not account for the many unmeasured and unknown variables presented by each individual.

Despite the difficulty of discussing your prognosis with your doctors, it's important that you do so. By understanding the "big picture," including the best and worst-case scenarios, you will be better able to make informed decisions about your treatment path.

Cure Versus Progression-Free Survival

Some brain tumors, like certain meningiomas and most pituitary tumors, are cured through surgery. Once surgically removed, these tumors never recur, even in the absence of additional treatment.

Progression-free survival is a difficult concept to grasp but an important one to understand as you contemplate various treatments. Most of us are familiar with cancer of the lung, breast, or other organs, where early detection can lead to an improved prognosis and lengthened survival rates. Such is not the case for primary brain tumors. Tumors that grow within the brain are intertwined with important brain cells. These neurons and axons are imperative to our daily activities of thinking, sensing, moving, and feeling. Because of this proximity, the removal of an entire brain tumor may be impossible without damage to functional cells nearby, a cause of permanent neurologic disability. Without the removal of the entire tumor, primary brain tumors eventually recur; the cancerous cells left in the brain continue to divide and grow. As a result, the concept of "cure" cannot accurately be applied.

"Neurologic progression-free survival" is a term in increasing use in clinical trials. It describes the likelihood a particular treatment will extend the time a person can live without neurological symptoms, such as weakness or language difficulties, even if that treatment cannot improve overall survival. For example, an individual might live 20 years after a diagnosis of a low-grade astrocytoma. Without treatment, he or she might experience a weak arm, a symptom of the growing tumor, at year 10 and endure that weakness for another 10 years. With treatment, that arm weakness might be delayed for another 2 or 5 years, reducing the patient's overall disability.

Average Overall Survival Versus Percentage of Long-Term Survivors

Statistics can help us understand how long the average person might expect to live given a certain treatment. But who is that average person? The average person is, unfortunately, no more than a compilation of past research data—not made of flesh and blood. More useful data might include the following: What are the characteristics of long-term survivors? And how many of them have been treated aggressively—with surgery, radiation therapy, and chemotherapy? Still, any answer to this last question might contain its own bias: indeed, it's possible that patients with the best prognostic factors are more likely to undergo aggressive therapy.

Without a doubt, it is important for you to find out the rough statistical information for your particular situation. Nevertheless, because so many variables go into a prognosis, you should try to avoid the impulse to "circle a date on the calendar." You are a unique individual in a unique medical situation. What's more, much of the recent brain tumor research invites cautious optimism. Discussions about prognosis are best had with your medical team over the course of your treatment and follow-up. As members of your care team get to know you better—and vice versa—and as they examine you and review your imaging results over time, the information about your prognosis will become clearer.

Time to Take Charge

By now you've been introduced to the basics about brain anatomy, common neurologic symptoms, and the various tests performed to make an accurate diagnosis. You may also have come to appreciate just how complicated this disease and its treatments can be. And you've begun to see how many people will touch your life as you go about making decisions regarding your care. Now is a good time to begin a record of your care, in hard copy or electronically. It need not be more complicated than a notebook or a computer folder where you can keep copies of all your documents. Be sure to ask your doctors to provide you with copies of the following:

- Consultation notes
  - Progress notes
  - Hospital discharge summaries
  - Operative reports
  - CT and MRI reports
- Pathology reports

It's helpful to keep this information in chronological order and to separate it into the categories listed earlier. Some hospitals record the discussion at tumor board, a meeting of physicians who discuss as a group the appropriate treatment for patients with cancer, taking care to consider all treatment options. If your hospital records these tumor board meetings, ask for a copy of the meeting where your particular situation was discussed. Also, keep copies of your imaging studies. These are, by law, housed in the radiology file room of the institution where the scans were taken (unlike the paper records mentioned previously, which are accessed through the medical records department of your hospital or clinic).

Ask your doctors to help you obtain a release of information form for this data, so you can keep it in one place. You may have to make a specific request for the actual CD holding your MRI images, or you're likely to receive only the paper report.

Your ability to get a second (or third) opinion will be improved if you keep your records on hand, organized, and at the ready.

Chapter 3

Understanding Radiation Therapy

Chris, a survivor of oligoastrocytoma of the right temporal lobe since 1996, marvels at the resiliency of his brain and of brains in general. After both the tumor and then the radiation therapy treatment caused memory loss, "I literally had to learn to retrain my brain," he says. "Other regions of my mind have taken over that short-term memory job that cancer destroyed. It's an amazing turnaround."

His body's resiliency inspires similar wonder. After undergoing a Gamma Knife procedure one Friday in December, he went hiking and fishing in the Cascade Mountains the following Sunday and Monday. Hesitant at first to take risks while undergoing treatment, he was inspired by the words of his neuro-oncologist: Get out there and live your life. "I took that to heart, started doing it, and I haven't stopped yet," he says.

Common treatment for primary brain tumors often includes radiation therapy, also known as radiotherapy. The therapy uses high-energy **ionizing radiation**, literally radioactive X-rays or gamma rays directed to the tumor site, to damage the cells' ability to multiply, which causes cell death. As the body eliminates the dead cells, the tumor will appear to stop growing or shrink on computerized tomography (CT) or magnetic resonance imaging (MRI) scans. The energy involved in radiation therapy is much higher than that used in diagnostic X-rays, such as CT scans and chest X-rays. As a result, radiation therapy can damage the surrounding normal brain tissue. However, healthy cells are resilient and with time are able to repair the damage.

Radiation therapy is delivered through two primary ways: external beam or internal, also known as **brachytherapy**. **External beam radiation therapy,** by far the most common form, uses an external source such as a **linear accelerator** to generate and direct radiation to the tumor or target. Internal radiation takes the form of radioactive seeds or liquids, which are implanted or injected directly into the brain tumor or surgical site.

In this chapter, you will learn the following:

- **How radiation therapy works**
- **The difference between external beam and internal radiation therapy**
- **The members of your radiation therapy team**
- **How long typical treatments last and what they are like**
- **The common side effects of radiation therapy**

Members of the Radiation Oncology Team

The radiation oncology team is made up of many highly trained professionals. Doctors who advise and oversee radiation therapy are known as radiation oncologists. Radiation therapists are the technicians who patients see each day of their therapy; they are certified to operate the treatment machines, such as the linear accelerators. Radiation oncology nurses provide patient education and help with symptom management. Medical physicists help ensure the treatment machines are calibrated and working properly; although they are a critical part of the treatment team, they do all of their work "behind the scenes" and are rarely seen by the patient. **Dosimetrists** help decide on beam angles, orientation, and weighting to come up with the desired treatment plan. Social workers and nutritionists also help patients recover well and remain symptom free.

Options for Primary Brain Tumors

There are several forms of external beam radiation therapy. The most common form is **three-dimensional conformal radiation therapy** (3D-CRT). 3D-CRT directs multiple radiation beams from various angles to deliver the desired dose to the tumor while avoiding the normal surrounding brain tissues or critical structures. Focusing each radiation beam to the tumor minimizes exposure to nearby organs and other areas of the brain. Figure 3–1 shows a typical planning study for radiation therapy of a brain tumor.

Preparing for Three-Dimensional Conformal Radiation Therapy

The planning phase may require two to three separate appointments before treatment can begin. At the first appointment, the patient is fitted with an **aquaplast mask**. This mask is made of a plastic mesh material that is pliable when soaked in warm water yet becomes rigid as it cools. It is used to immobilize the patient's head and face while, of course, permitting breathing and minor movement. Once in the mask and lying down in the treatment position, the patient then undergoes what is known as a treatment-planning CT scan. This process, called simulation, helps determine the optimal head position during 3D-CRT treatment and takes about 30 to 60 minutes. The patient's prior recent CT or MRI may be used as ancillary studies to aid treatment planning.

Next, the radiation oncologist will contour, or chart out, the area that needs to be treated, along with other brain structures. The radiation oncologist works with the dosimetrist (a member of the radiation therapy team trained in the calculation and technical issues concerning the dose of treatment) and the physicist to come up with the most effective beam arrangement and

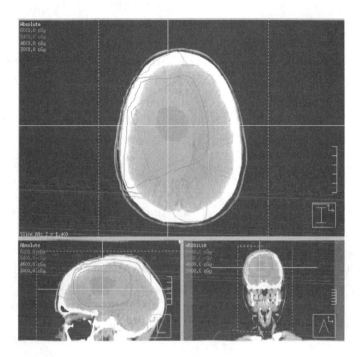

FIGURE 3-1 Radiation therapy. Three different views of a computed tomographic (CT) planning study of a brain tumor (red), swelling around the tumor (green), and treatment lines for radiation therapy shown in axial (lying down) view, side view, and front view.

blocking pattern to deliver the dose to the tumor while minimizing impact to other brain structures. Often, when treating an infiltrative process like a glioma, a rim of normal brain tissue surrounding the tumor will intentionally be treated to target all areas where tumor tentacles are suspected to exist. This exacting process takes place largely behind the scenes in the weeks following surgery. It will often take 2 to 3 weeks to perfect the treatment. During this time, many patients and their family members become anxious about perceived delays. Be patient! This time is very important to making sure that the radiation therapy is perfectly individualized.

Once the plan is completed, the patient comes back for a "dry test run," otherwise called a field verification or "simulation." This process takes about 30 to 45 minutes and is done in the treatment room. The patient is set up on the treatment table as if to receive treatment, but instead all the beams and blocking patterns are checked for accuracy. Once the match is solid, the patient then is given a time to start the treatment. Typical 3D-CRT treatments are given daily (Monday through Friday) over a period of 5 to 7 weeks. Each daily treatment, called a fraction, lasts about 15 minutes.

During treatment, some people notice an odd smell caused by the ozone produced by the linear accelerator, and some patients may also see colored lights behind their eyes. Such symptoms are common and nothing to be worried about. In fact, they can help you visualize the radiation therapy damaging the tumor.

Important Considerations

In treating anything as challenging as a brain tumor, consistency and timeliness are the name of the game. Although the dosages and associated therapies will vary depending on tumor type, some words of wisdom apply uniformly.

(1) Because radiation therapy requires daily treatments over a span of 6 weeks in one geographic location, choose a location that offers the best treatment possible as well as high levels of caregiver support, as the daily drive is not likely to be one you can do by yourself.

(2) Plan to complete the treatment within the designated time frame, as delays, such as taking a week or two off in the middle, may reduce its efficacy.

(3) Complete the therapy at the same treatment facility. Different facilities tend to have different equipment, and transferring care to another facility will often require starting anew with the treatment planning, which may cause interruptions in treatment. In addition, it may be difficult to get an accurate overall dose because essentially two different plans will need to be summated, or added together.

Dosage Specifics

For high-grade tumors: A standard dose for a malignant or high-grade glioma is 60 gray (Gy). A gray is an absorbed dose of radiation. Each tissue in the body has a maximum lifetime dose of radiation that is considered to be safe. Sixty gray has proven to be the best dose for treating brain tumors, but it is also at the upper limit; once radiation therapy has been completed, no further doses can be given, with the exception of those through stereotactic radiosurgery, discussed later (see "Retreatment"). Higher doses have been tested in clinical trials but have not shown any significant improvement in survival rates and are associated with a higher risk of side effects, such as a skin rash like sunburn, fatigue, swelling of the tumor or memory loss several years after the completion of the treatment. For glioblastoma multiforme (GBM), a chemotherapy drug, **temozolomide (Temodar)**, is also taken daily during the 6 weeks of radiation therapy; it is thought to act as a "radiosensitizer" because it makes the tumor cells more receptive to the effects of radiation therapy. Once completed, the patient will enjoy a 4-week break and then resume temozolomide therapy. The addition of temozolomide has been shown to improve the chance of survival for GBM compared to the survival seen with radiation therapy alone.

For low-grade tumors: The standard dose for low-grade gliomas is 54 Gy. The treatment is delivered over 5 to 6 weeks in 27 to 30 fractions.

Other External Beam Radiation Therapies

A recent advance in the delivery of radiation is **intensity-modulated radiation therapy (IMRT)**. IMRT differs from 3D-CRT in its ability to modify the intensity of the radiation within each radiation beam. As a result, this treatment is able to calibrate the radiation dosage by the size and shape of the treatment fields and the size and shape of the tumor. Compared to 3D-CRT, it takes longer to deliver a fraction each day, 20 to 30 minutes compared to 10 to 15 minutes. The technique may be useful for tumors that are close to critical organs, such as eyes or nerves, or with well-delineated borders such as meningiomas. In general, it does not offer any advantage over 3D-CRT in treating infiltrative tumors such as gliomas.

Stereotactic radiotherapy (SRT), or **stereotactic radiosurgery (SRS)**, pinpoints high doses of radiation directly on the tumor, in some cases in only one treatment. The tumor is located with bull's-eye accuracy through reference markers on a head frame or implanted in the patient's skull. Such treatment may be useful in treating small tumors, such as metastasis (tumors that have spread from other parts of the body to the brain), meningiomas (a common benign tumor), or other small, well-defined tumors. However, this treatment is not appropriate as "first-line" therapy for infiltrative processes such as gliomas, although in rare cases, it may be useful for treating small **recurrent** gliomas. Linear accelerators can be adapted to deliver SRT or SRS. With a linear accelerator, multiple or single fractions can be given. For single-fraction treatment, the patient will likely wear a head frame to immobilize the skull. In multiple-fraction treatments, an aquaplastic mask or bite-block system, like a panorama X-ray at the dentist office, is used.

The **Gamma Knife**, a machine specially designed for radiosurgery, provides treatment in a single fraction with pinpoint accuracy. The treatment uses gamma radiation emitted from radioactive cobalt sources within the unit. The patient wears a head frame that is affixed to his or her skull with two screws in the front and two in the back. While the patient undergoes an MRI of the brain, permanent reference markers on the head frame allow for the tumor's precise stereotactic localization. Typically, planning for the treatment and the actual treatment itself occur the same day.

Proton therapy is similar to external beam therapy, except it uses a proton particle instead of X-rays to kill brain tumor cells. Currently, it remains rare and is available in only a few treatment centers in the United States. Protons have a property called the Bragg peak, which describes a steep gradient in the buildup and drop-off of the dose deposited in the tissue. In other words, protons are able to deposit a dose of treatment in the desired area with very little deposited in the tissues surrounding the tumor. This precision may be an advantage when treating tumors close to critical organs, such as the eyes and the optic nerves, and in children, whose developing brains must be protected from unnecessary radiation.

Brachytherapy, or the surgical implantation of radiation energy into or near a tumor, has been used for brain tumors but with limited success. Requiring special training to perform, it is more frequently used to treat tumors that have recurred, often in conjunction with surgery. During this treatment, a closed-end catheter or tube is inserted into the brain, through which a radioactive substance or a strand of radioactive seeds is injected. Patients must stay in the hospital for a few days during this treatment. Once treatment is complete, the radioactive substance is withdrawn. Another method is to permanently place radioactive sources into the tumor during surgery.

Side Effects of Radiation Therapy

Peggy, whose treatment for grade 3 oligoastrocytoma of the left frontal lobe included radiation therapy, found the fatigue and everydayness of it particularly "grueling." Yet the loss of her straight blond hair truly unnerved her. "Something as simple as

*hair loss is not that simple," she says. "A lot of my feminine iden-
tity is wrapped up in my hair. Now it's growing in weird, gray and
curly. Wearing a scarf every day is a pain in the butt. I'm more
self-conscious."*

Every treatment has its side effects, and radiation therapy is no
different. Prior to treatment, the radiation oncologist or nurse will
review possible side effects with the patient and caregiver; during
treatment, patients will meet with the radiation oncologist at least
weekly to address symptom management. Most patients notice
greater side effects as the therapy proceeds. For instance, during a
6-week course of 3D-CRT, a patient may begin to notice side effects
after the second or third week, and most acutely in the final week,
or even the week after the therapy ends.

The most common acute side effects are fatigue, hair loss, and
scalp or skin irritation, much like sunburn. Less common side
effects include headaches, nausea, dry eyes, nasal congestion, and
a change in appetite. Many side effects can be treated with medications and are fleeting. Fatigue and skin and scalp irritation will
improve within weeks following therapy. Light or moderate exercise with adequate rest may help reduce fatigue. The skin/scalp may
become darker and peel similar to the healing of sunburn. Because
the scalp will become more sensitive to the sun, it is important
to keep a hat handy during activity outdoors. A variety of topical
medications, such as aloe vera and hydrocortisone, will help calm
skin or scalp irritation. Nevertheless, during radiation therapy
patients should consult their radiation oncologist before applying
any product to the skin.

Other side effects may be longer lasting. For instance, hair
may take several months to grow back, may be thinner, and
may have different characteristics—such as appearing curlier or
straighter—than before treatment. If the ear canals are in the
treatment area, swollen tissues near the tumor site may cause
muffled hearing or ear congestion; over-the-counter nasal or sinus

decongestants (e.g., Afrin, Sudafed) frequently relieve such symptoms. Although usually temporary, on rare occasion a permanent decrease in hearing can result. Headaches and nausea may occur due to brain swelling from the radiation or the tumor. Headaches can be treated with pain medications and/or oral corticosteroids, such as dexamethasone, which help reduce the brain swelling. In the event of significant nausea, patients may need prescription antinausea medications. Brain swelling may also cause symptoms that mimic those of the brain tumor, such as muscle weakness or speech difficulties.

Some side effects from radiation therapy may occur or become noticeable months after treatment. Such effects most often result from alterations in the blood supply to the irradiated area of the brain. Late effects commonly include swelling or brain edema, which can cause headaches and other stroke-like symptoms. Radiation necrosis, which describes an area of normal brain tissue that has died and formed scar tissue, is rare but may also occur; this condition can often be confused with a recurrent brain tumor. Steroids are useful in both treating brain edema and radiation necrosis and relieving their related symptoms. However, sometimes surgery may be required to remove this dead tissue.

Finally, some side effects from radiation therapy, like seizures and hormonal imbalances, can be alarming. If the pituitary gland is in the treatment field, radiation therapy may alter normal hormone levels, leading to thyroid problems or troubles with sugar metabolism, infertility, or an inability to process water. Such hormonal imbalances can be diagnosed by blood tests and treated with medications under the care of an endocrinologist. Other side effects include a slowing down of cognitive function, affecting memory and the ability to perform calculations. Attention and concentration can sometimes be affected as well. Drugs used to treat attention deficit disorders, such as methylphenidate (more commonly known as Ritalin) can be of help.

Retreatment

When a tumor recurs, or starts growing again, many patients will ask about the possibility of undergoing additional radiation therapy. Many factors go into such a decision, including the prior dose given to the patient, the area and amounts of brain previously treated, how long ago the last radiation treatment was given, and the size and location of the recurrent or new tumor. Side effects are another important consideration. Once the patient has received a full course (60 Gy) of radiation therapy to the brain, any subsequent radiation therapy may elevate the risk of side effects, such as those previously mentioned. As a result, the risks of additional treatment often outweigh its benefits. However, in rare situations of a small, localized recurrence, SRS or SRT may continue to be an option.

Radiation Therapy for Brain Metastases

Because brain metastases are tumors that begin in another location (breast, lung, kidney, for example), then spread to the brain through the blood supply, treatment of the whole brain with radiation therapy is often performed to ensure that microscopic tumors are completely treated. **Whole-brain radiotherapy (WBRT)** is typically given to a dose of 30 Gy—37.5 Gy over 2–3 weeks instead of the partial brain treatment given in 60 Gy over 6 weeks, as earlier discussed. A concern among patients and doctors is growing over the possible side effects of significant memory loss from whole-brain radiotherapy. As a result, single metastases are increasingly being treated with SRS or SRT; however, this remains a controversial approach as many neuro-oncologists believe there is a higher risk of tumor growth outside the small SRS field. Surgical removal of single brain metastases is often preferred, but only when the disease in the rest of the body is under control.

Radiation Therapy for Meningioma, Acoustic Neuroma, and Pituitary Adenoma

Meningiomas, acoustic neuromas, and pituitary adenomas are most likely to require radiation therapy when they have been incompletely removed, have recurred after surgical removal, or are growing at the base of the skull close to important structures. Rarely, these tumors may be malignant or have aggressive features that can invade the brain. In this situation, radiation therapy is recommended even if there is complete removal of the tumor. In such cases, they are best treated with Gamma Knife, IMRT, or SRS/SRT procedures.

PART 2

How Do I Deal with This?

Chapter 4

Lifestyle Management

People do a lot of things when faced with a cancer diagnosis. Cry. Eat. Grieve. Swear. Fret. All of these responses are perfectly natural. But some people funnel that energy into activity.

Shiy was pregnant with her fourth child when she was diagnosed with an anaplastic astrocytoma. A fan of Pilates and of exercise in general, she was anything but a couchsitter. So, after the baby's birth, and upon completion of chemotherapy, she pulled out her running shoes. "I just contacted one of my friends and asked if she wanted to run," she says "I want to do a marathon before I die. That's my new goal."

Lack of control is one of the most common feelings when people are faced with a cancer diagnosis. It makes sense: you didn't choose the disease—it found you. Fortunately, exercise, nutrition, and stress reduction are three pursuits through which you can restore some sense of power. What's more, many people find comfort in considering the use of natural or holistic remedies. What follows are some general recommendations about ways you can continue to live your life, feel good, and most of all, feel like yourself. But before you set off on any new exercise or diet regimen, or pick up where you left off, make sure to discuss it with your doctor.

In this chapter, you will learn the following:

- **How deep breathing and meditation can relieve stress and improve well-being**

- The importance of maintaining a healthy diet and ways to begin eating better
- Why exercise continues to be important during your recovery
- Current thinking about complementary alternative therapies, including herbal and dietary supplements
- The challenges—and opportunities—when you have to break from driving
- The value of support groups for some people
- Ways to cope with hair loss and changes to your appearance
- How creative pursuits can be personally enriching

Feel Empowered

There's no denying that a brain tumor diagnosis will shake your world and, quite possibly, your view of yourself within it. Once the trips to the doctors begin, the hair begins to thin, and the label "cancer patient" starts to stick, many people find themselves bearing up as a "tragic victim" of the disease, a "brave soldier" fighting against it, or a "heroic caregiver" where once they were just a spouse, a sibling, a friend. Convenient for others, these roles may come up short in describing the complexity of your feelings.

Here's the thing to remember: You are not your tumor. Your tumor doesn't own you. You are you, and you also have a serious medical condition for which you or your loved one is being treated. That's where empowerment comes in. Empowerment is not simply putting a smile on one's face under the impression that a positive outlook will produce miracles. Instead, it means concentrating on what you truly value, your core source of peace and strength, and seeking ways to bring more of that into your life.

Astrid Pujari, MD, operates the Pujari Center, a clinic that integrates Western and holistic medicine in Seattle, WA. She is a board-certified internist and credentialed medical herbalist who treats many people dealing with cancer (and has contributed many insights to this chapter). She urges her patients to try to answer these questions: Who am I really? Why am I alive? Who am I living for? What do I value? What brings me a sense of love, peace, and connection? What can I do to invite more of those things in my life? Your answers might surprise you—and they may suggest new places to put your energy. "Ironically," Dr. Pujari says, many patients "feel more alive now than ever before because they start paying attention to what matters to them."

Dr. Pujari also suggests this empowerment exercise: Think back to a specific time or event when you have felt at peace or connected to others. Now, spending a few moments with your eyes closed, reconstruct that experience in as much detail as possible. "Imagine that experience growing, swelling, flowing into your feet, hands, gut, head," she says. "Feel that feeling and enlarge it. Then imagine doing things where you literally, intentionally, start with that feeling."

Reduce Stress

Reducing stress during trying times is often easier said than done. Our lives can feel stressful and overpacked even in the best of times. Nevertheless, for our bodies to be most receptive to treatment and focus on healing, it's important to minimize stress and increase relaxation.

A well-balanced life depends on three factors: emotional, spiritual, and mental health.

(1) Emotional health refers to the effects of stress on health through the sympathetic nervous system. Mind/body techniques such as prayer, meditation, breathing, yoga, biofeedback, and regular exercise can decrease those physical effects of stress. Focused breathing techniques are also

helpful, as is mindfulness, a technique that emphasizes the ins and outs of each individual breath and the circumstances of the moment over the constant clutter of outside stimuli.

(2) Mental health refers to the effects of brain chemistry and its ability to alter mood. Patients who have cancer sometimes feel symptoms of depression, such as fatigue, loss of appetite, diminished concentration, loss of energy, and a reduced sex drive. As someone who has been on the receiving end of a brain tumor diagnosis, you and your caregiver have every right to feel sad, a sense of loss, or even anger. Feel free to discuss these feelings with your doctor. However, if they persist and keep you from being able to function fully, you may benefit from counseling and/or medication. Similarly, sleep disturbance is common for those undergoing tumor treatments, and it can also be a sign of depression.

A few recommendations for a good night's sleep:

- Go to bed and wake up at the same time each day. A sleep routine cues your body rhythms for rest.
- Reserve your bed for sleeping and sex. That means avoiding taking your laptop, newspapers, and TV to bed with you, which can signal the mind to stay active just when you want it to wind down.
- Keep the room cool (68 to 72 degrees) and dark.
- Avoid caffeinated beverages, exercise, and alcohol in the evening.
- Consider daily meditation to declutter your mind before bed.
- If sleepless nights persist, discuss the use of a sedative with your doctor.

(3) Spiritual health refers to all the things that give life a sense of meaning and help us get out of bed each morning. While we're focusing on restoring physical health, it's easy to neglect some of these other aspects of our lives. Whether it comes from nurturing our children, walking the dog, praying to a higher power, connecting with friends, or watching the sunset each day, spiritual health helps us maintain our energy and interest in life.

Breathe Deeply

We all know that breathing delivers oxygen to our lungs, which forces it throughout our bodies along the red blood cell superhighway. Though it is necessary to life, breathing is hardly a constant. When we're sound asleep, our breathing is smooth and steady (unless we have sleep apnea, when it tends to be erratic). After we run, we gasp for air. When we watch scary movies, our breathing grows shallower and quicker. When we're nervous, the agitated puffs of breath we take tend not to make it deep into our diaphragm. As a result, our emotions can control our breath, and likewise, our breath can control our emotions.

If you want to feel calmer, all you need to do is to take a few deep breaths. In three breaths, you can slow down your heart rate and think more clearly. As Dr. Pujari says, "For most people, what's difficult about disease is controlling their emotions about it. So how do we empower people? Before you go to your doctor's appointment, take three deep breaths. Or if you want to be in a more loving space with someone, take three breaths."

Consider Meditation

Recent studies have shown the many positive benefits of meditation to help focus and clarify your thoughts. But did you know meditation is also linked to physical benefits, such as reduced blood pressure and heart rate, lower rates of depression, and improved operations of your healing and nervous systems? It may be easy to dismiss this ancient practice as just an excuse for sitting around chanting "om." Yet individuals who meditate for just 10 minutes a day report a long list of positive impacts, backed by research data.

Types of Meditation

According to Dr. Pujari, three forms of meditation show proven physical and psychological benefits:

- Mindfulness meditation: Based in Buddhist practice, this form has you focused on noticing each breath coming in and out of your body for 3 or more minutes.
- Transcendental meditation: Based in Indian spirituality, this form requires formal teaching and involves the repetition of a mantra or special word.
- Guided imagery meditation: This form asks you to visualize an event or experience before it happens.

These brief overviews hardly do justice to a practice that has been popular since before the Buddha ("enlightened one") sat beneath the Bodhi tree. If you'd like to learn more, there are countless books, CDs, DVDs, Web sites, and community classes across the country dedicated to the topic and each particular meditation form.

Move Your Muscles

Perhaps you're a natural athlete, always up for physical activity. Or maybe you look for ways to fit long walks, tennis matches, yoga, or swimming laps into your daily or weekly routine. Or maybe you'd prefer doing just about anything to moving your muscles. No matter your approach, exercise may not be at the top of your list depending on where you are in the cycle of your diagnosis and treatment. Nevertheless, increasing your heart rate for 30 minutes most days of the week has proven health benefits. A goal of 30 minutes may seem steep, but it is only a goal. A good place to start might be a walk around the neighborhood, or even just out to the mailbox. If you belong to a gym, you might want to consult with a personal trainer about a light exercise program. Some people have the strength and stamina to run marathons. Others celebrate the victory of a few steps outside for some fresh air. Wherever your starting point is, just start and don't give up.

Eat Well

Maintaining a healthful diet, much less a healthy appetite, can be difficult while undergoing treatments for cancer. Because of the changes your body is undergoing, food may not be as appetizing as it once was. What's more, the process of radiation and the use of chemotherapy drugs will cause some foods to taste different—making favorite foods less flavorful, or leaving a metallic taste in your mouth—but this should improve in time. Nonetheless, to maintain your strength, you'll need to eat.

This quick list reflects some basics about nutrition and will likely yield few surprises. The items mentioned here are healthful for everyone, including patient, caregiver, and children.

(1) Increase your intake of fresh fruits and vegetables; 10 servings a day is ideal.
(2) Drink plenty of water, at least eight 8 oz. glasses a day. During treatment, it can be easy to become dehydrated.
(3) Choose brown things instead of white things (e.g., whole grain rice, bread, pasta) to increas e your intake of fiber and

B vitamins, both of which aid digestion and the immune system.

(4) Eat more healthy, monounsaturated fats such as olive oil and omega-3 oils from fish like sardines, anchovies, mackerel, salmon, and halibut. You can also use fish oil supplements (see list later in this chapter).

(5) Eat less saturated fat, found in red meats and dairy products, and partially hydrogenated oils—so-called trans fats—frequently found in processed and fast foods.

(6) During chemo and radiation therapy, increase your intake of protein from nuts, kale, Swiss chard, and other sources.

(7) Avoid refined white sugar, especially high-fructose corn syrup—unless that slice of birthday cake will make you over-the-moon happy, then be sure to savor every bite!

Alcohol

During brain radiation treatment, it is wise to limit alcohol intake to one glass of beer or wine with dinner, if at all. Heavy consumption of alcohol can increase the likelihood of seizures or interact with your antiseizure medications, slowing down memory and making you unsteady on your feet. The advice really isn't so different from what you've heard before: moderation rules, and abstaining reigns supreme. Also, make sure to follow any dietary restrictions associated with certain medications.

> A former Peace Corps volunteer turned lawyer, Paul is open to unexpected sources of wisdom, but he also always consults his doctor about any alternative medicines or therapies he considers taking—like ginger, which is associated with many anticancer and anti-inflammatory benefits. "I'd consider alternative medicines," he says. "I don't think Western practitioners have the sole answer. They have an answer."

Herbal and Dietary Supplements

Patients often ask about the benefits of certain dietary supplements, vitamins, herbal treatments, and other natural remedies. Without a doubt, many botanical agents offer effective treatments, *with this caveat*: They must be used under medical supervision, just like a prescription drug. Many holistic treatments contain medicinal properties that might interact—both positively and negatively—with drugs and treatments prescribed by your doctors. For instance, some supplements (e.g., St. John's Wort) can cause photosensitivity; their effects may be compounded during radiation therapy and cause extreme skin discomfort. Some enhance metabolism, thereby weakening the effectiveness of certain drugs. Others thin the blood, making surgery hazardous if their use isn't terminated weeks in advance. To ensure the best possible outcome, please discuss any use of such products with your care team as well as with an experienced herbal practitioner.

If you do choose to integrate herbal and dietary supplements into your regimen, make sure you get what you're paying for. Many supplements available online or sold over the counter are neither regulated nor approved for use by the US Food and Drug Administration (FDA). As a result, they may not contain the ingredients stated on the label or in the quantities promised. Dr. Pujari recommends purchasing supplements from manufacturers that have been certified by the United States Pharmacopeia (USP), a nonprofit public health organization that sets standards for prescription and over-the-counter medicines and other health care products manufactured or sold in the United States (http://www.usp.org). Another resource is http://www.consumerlab.com, a company that independently tests the quality and efficacy of health and nutritional products, but its results are available by subscription only.

Following are several dietary supplements you may want to consider. For detailed information about these and others, go to the Integrative Medicine section of the Memorial Sloan-Kettering Cancer Center Web site.

(1) Multivitamins: Chemotherapy and radiation can curb appetite, making it difficult to get proper nutrition. Consider taking a daily multivitamin that provides 100 percent of US required daily allowances (USRDA). Be sure to avoid taking more than you need as your system may already be strained.

(2) Vitamin D: Found in some epidemiological studies to decrease the risk for developing cancer, vitamin D also helps with bone growth and boosts immune system cells. Though it is a natural benefit of sunlight, your skin is unlikely to absorb enough vitamin D without also inviting serious sun damage. Absorption rates depend on many factors, including where you live (sunny Arizona vs. gray Seattle), your complexion, level of outdoor activity, and age. Look for vitamin D in gels, capsules, or liquids, optimally in its natural (vitamin D3) form, which is more effective. Many experts recommend 2,000 international units (IU) per day, though you may want to have your current levels tested first.

(3) Fish oil: For optimal health, the human body needs two oils—omega-3 (from fats found in fish as well as flaxseed and hempseed oil) and omega-6 (found in nearly every other oil). To decrease inflammation in the body and to improve immune-system response, consider taking a supplement containing omega-3. However, daily consumption of more than 3 grams of omega-3 oil may increase the risk of bleeding, especially if you're taking common blood thinners (e.g., coumadin, warfarin, or heparin). Again, be sure to discuss the use of this and any supplement with your medical care team.

(4) Green tea: Studies have shown that people who have a higher consumption rate of green tea have a lower risk of cancer of all types, though whether that's because of the green tea itself or a host of other variables is unknown. Nonetheless, green

tea has won many champions. Using fresher, "greener" leaves than traditional black teas, green tea contains epigallocatechin gallate (EGCG), an antioxidant thought to be beneficial in treating certain cancer types. Other attributed benefits include the prevention of cellular damage and a decrease in new blood vessel growth to cancer cells. A couple of downsides to green tea exist. It may interfere with blood-thinning regimens, and the caffeinated form may interfere with sleep. Green tea is also available in capsules.

(5) Turmeric: An herbal root from the ginger family, tumeric contains the pigment curcumin, an antioxidant that has been shown to promote the death of cancer cells and also has anti-inflammatory properties. Turmeric is best when consumed in capsule form with a fat-soluble base (or eaten in huge quantities, which is not advised). Turmeric has few side effects and tends to be very well tolerated.

(6) Resveratrol: This plant pigment, found in the skin of red grapes, is believed to have anti-inflammatory, antioxidant, and anticancer properties. A flavonoid, or active plant compound, resveratrol also provides the heart-healthy and digestive benefits of alcohol without the need for heavy consumption. Talk to an expert about optimal dosage and possible medicinal side effects.

Driving

John, a resident of Mill Creek, WA, has been living with a cerebellar astrocytoma since 1995. At the time of his diagnosis, his two daughters were on the cusp of that teenage rite: learning to drive. John vowed to be part of it. "When I was first diagnosed, I told the doctor, 'Make me good so I can teach my daughters how to drive.'" Having accomplished that goal, the lifelong car lover now wields a transit pass with a similar pride. "I went to training on

*how to ride the bus with my daughter," he says, charting a course
for a future of bus-schedule reading and route transfers. "Now I
teach everyone I know how to ride the bus."*

From a very early age, many of us view driving as a symbol
of freedom, independence, and self-sufficiency. Indeed, because
of modern society's emphasis on the car, it can be difficult *not* to
drive. Yet many people diagnosed with brain tumors are faced with
just that. Because of the complex motor functions driving requires,
they can no longer drive safely—for the safety of themselves, their
passengers, and fellow motorists and pedestrians. For a while, and
perhaps longer, you may need to rely on others and public transit
to get around.

Later, your driving abilities can be reevaluated by computer
program and by occupational therapists. Some states offer active
disabled driving programs that will allow you to drive with a rehabilitation therapist. However, if you are experiencing active seizures with a loss of consciousness, most states will not legally allow
you to drive for 6 months and sometimes longer. Check with your
local department of motor vehicles for your state's rules.

Signs that you should hang up your keys:

(1) State laws: Check the local Department of Motor Vehicles (DMV)
     Web site or ask your doctor about any state driving restrictions
     you need to heed. To drive well requires quick reflexes, good
     peripheral vision, eye-hand coordination, and hand and foot
     strength. Depending on the type of tumor you have, your agil-
     ity affecting those areas may not be what it once was.

(2) A recent history of seizures: Every state has rules regarding
     when drivers can return to the road after a seizure, varying
     from 6 months to 2 years. Driving restrictions reset with
     each generalized seizure causing a loss of consciousness
     and apply regardless of whether you are taking antiseizure
     medications.

(3) Concern of your passengers: Family members and friends are often good early barometers for your driving safety. If your passengers feel unsafe, discuss driving with your doctor and consider doing specialized testing, which in many states is provided by a comprehensive rehabilitation program. Specially trained driving rehabilitation providers will drive in your car with you and specifically test you for neurologic skills required in driving, such as speed of information processing, language variables, and judgment. This is often expensive testing but worth it in the long run if there is any doubt about your abilities.

Many occupational therapists can do a quick computer-based driving screen for safety, and many on-the-road evaluation programs, some specifically geared toward the medically impaired driver, are available. Departments of rehabilitation medicine in large academic medical centers are a good place to start, as is a consultation with a physiatrist (rehabilitation medicine physician), physical therapist, or occupational therapist.

Early on in the treatment process, getting to radiation therapy appointments without driving can be a logistical hurdle. As you read in Chapter 3: Understanding Radiation Therapy, treatments take place daily during the week, with weekends off, over a course of 3 to 7 weeks, depending on tumor type. Such frequency will require a resourceful approach; however, once the word is out, you might be surprised to see all those willing to play chauffeur. This simple but necessary task can be an ideal opportunity for friends, family, and neighbors to show you their support. Having or being a "designated driver" for the day, when paired with a short outing like lunch, can be a small but welcome part of your recovery.

For those who live far from their treatment centers, many hospitals have hotel accommodations nearby to make the driving issue less burdensome. The American Cancer Society has a program to help defray hotel costs. Check with the cancer center social worker for details.

Working

During the first 3 months following a brain tumor diagnosis, you will be surrounded by new faces, new routines, new medications, new schedules, and the frequent juggling of appointments. In general, very few people, if they can help it, choose to work full time while undergoing treatment; radiation therapy alone takes up a part of each day (except for weekends) for 6 weeks.

Of course, much depends on the tumor type and location, treatment course (surgery vs. radiation therapy and chemotherapy, or a combination), and the severity of symptoms and side effects. Another variable is the nature of your job—a pilot may have more constraints than, perhaps, a paralegal or pet walker. Talk with your medical team about your particular situation and level of interest in resuming work.

Many people undergoing brain tumor treatment take a 3-month stay of short-term medical disability; it will allow you to focus on managing your treatment, reorganizing your priorities, and getting proper rest. You may also need to consider long-term disability; ask your doctor for a candid discussion of your prognosis so that you know what to expect during and after treatment.

Good sources of information about medical disability include hospital social workers and your employer's human resource department. Another source of help is the federal Family and Medical Leave Act (FMLA), which allows certain employees with up to 12 weeks of unpaid, job-protected leave per year. Federal disability programs are there for a reason—and, though our culture rewards hard work, your job now is to survive your illness and recuperate.

If you do decide to return to work, try to ease back in on a part-time basis to assess your strength and stamina. And remember: Only the rarest few of us will ever say, in our parting words, "I wish I had spent more time at work."

Support Groups

Many cancer centers host support groups, but few offer groups tailored exclusively for those living with brain tumors. Still, it's well worth the effort to try to find one, even if the group exists solely online. Typically facilitated by a nurse and a social worker, the meetings may begin with a short informational lecture by a health professional before breaking out into a more informal, social group. Attending one can help lift you up, provide education, laughter, energy, and a strong sense of community. Often it's the one place where you feel free to express your full gamut of emotions (including the negative and even dark ones that you shield from others) because you know that you are all united in a common purpose: to have the absolute best quality of life possible.

The National Brain Tumor Society and the American Association of Brain Tumors keep an updated list of support groups around the country; check online or call for a listing. If you live outside a major metropolitan area, your doctor should be able to suggest another patient who might be willing to talk by phone or correspond over the Internet. An ever-growing array of online chat groups can also be helpful. These days, community can be as close as your fingertips (Figure 4–1).

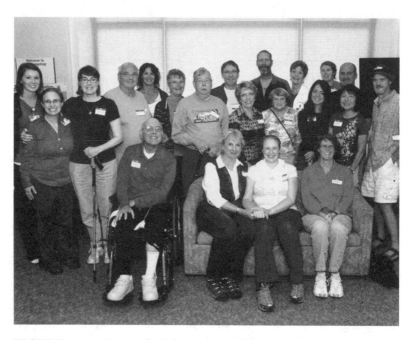

FIGURE 4–1 The wonderful Brain Tumor Support Group at Virginia Mason Medical Center, Seattle, Washington.

Cosmetic Issues

Peggy, who underwent treatment for a grade 3 oligodendro-glioma, said the loss of her blond locks sent her reeling. Coy's observation echoes many people's feelings when faced with changes they see in the mirror as a result of a brain tumor. "It was very traumatic to be in the shower and watch it come out," she says. Somehow, those strands circling the drain felt like a blow to her sense of self. Though she now wears a scarf daily, she calls it "a pain in the butt." Still, it's a concession she makes to fit in with a hair-focused society and to feel more herself.

Hair loss is likely for most people with brain tumors. Whether it results from the head being shaved in preparation for surgery or radiation therapy and/or chemotherapy—both of which can cause your hair to come out in clumps—chances are good your thick pelt, if you have one, will lose its luster, at least for a time. But don't despair—hair grows back!

A craniotomy scar is more difficult to conceal than a scar elsewhere on the body. Today, many neurosurgeons will accommodate a request to minimize the amount of shaving needed around the incision, allowing you to obscure the scar later with clever styling.

Hair loss from radiation therapy can be quite complete within the irradiated area, which covers the area of your tumor with some similar hair loss on the opposite side of your head. Oddly, hair often grows back in a different color or texture than what was there previously. Rates of hair growth are very individual, but you can generally expect it to take 6 months to a year.

> Serry had long hair her entire life. But that all changed when she was treated for medulloblastoma. When her hair started falling out, she had her head shaved. "I love being bald," she says. "Everybody keeps telling me I have a beautiful head. You have to be adaptable to your circumstances."

In the meantime, many female patients rush out to buy wigs, only to find them hot, itchy, and uncomfortable. Some do find choices that work for them, so shop around. It may be possible for your doctor to write a prescription for "hair prosthesis," allowing it to be covered by insurance. Others have found that letting the hair grow to a short length and then getting hair extensions works well for them. Scarves, hats, and baseball caps are other common solutions. So is going bald and proud.

Applying makeup can be difficult for people experiencing muscle weakness or tremors. If your style includes makeup, it's possible to get "permanent makeup," which includes cosmetic procedures that dye the eyebrows and eyelashes and ink eyeliner much like a tattoo.

Creativity, Art, and Humor as Therapy

Serry has been spinning wool for decades. That hasn't stopped, even though her foot strength has diminished during treatment for medullablastoma. "I like to have something I'm working on that's functional," she says. "The [spinning wheel] pedal is big enough for both of my feet. As soon as I move off the treadle, I can move my right foot a bit. It's soothing and relaxing."

When faced with a serious illness, some people rediscover creative outlets they once loved or plow their energy into new ones. They may find it soothing, or so consuming that it takes their minds off treatment for hours at a time. Either way, creativity is deeply affirming of people's core humanity, no matter what form it takes: writing, painting, drawing, knitting, spinning, cooking, sculpting, sewing, singing, quilting (Figure 4–2).

A daily private journal or an online blog for friends and families is a good place to start. Both work to focus your thoughts and harness energy for the treatments that lie ahead. Abundant research shows that when the left side of the brain is compromised by strokes, tumors, or dementia, the right side can actually become more creative. Using art as therapy, one can often express feelings difficult to express in words (Figure 4–3). Sometimes the tumor itself becomes the subject of the artwork. For instance, before an upcoming surgery, one potter threw 15 ceramic "tumor" pots. She then hosted a party, inviting the guests to "smash my tumor" with hammers. In the intensive care unit, she placed a carved "tumor board" at her bedside, consisting of a box with tiny figures of her

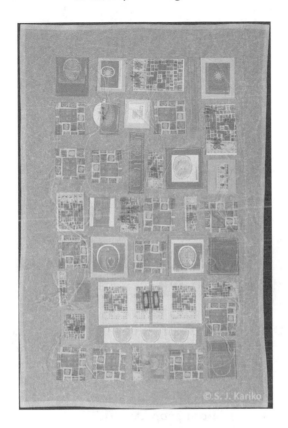

FIGURE 4-2 *Unobstructed View V.* Paper, magnetic resonance imaging (MRI) scans, hope, hinge, resilience, thread, beads, wire, love 30" x 22", 2009 by S. J. Kariko. Copyright © 2009 by S. J. Kariko. All rights reserved. Photo Credit: Neil Dixon, Yankee Imaging.

"In this piece, I manipulate pre- and post-operative (post-radiation but pre-chemo) MRI images of my husband's tennis-ball sized grade IV Glioblastoma multiforme. It hangs in our home—a daily reminder to dig deep into life everyday, and that for any of us, all we ever have is this very moment."

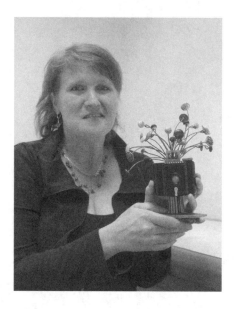

FIGURE 4-3 Sarah Hedman, a young woman with a glioma, pictured here with her artistic version of a brain. Sarah used her art to help her cope with her treatment and give it additional meaning.

neuro-oncologist, neurosurgeon, and pathologist. At every subsequent clinic visit, she presented a new creation, always focused on some aspect of living life with a brain tumor. It became a springboard for her to bring up difficult topics and an opportunity for her to own her illness and participate in her recovery.

Chapter 5

Symptom Management and Palliative Care

Palliative care is often thought to be the care given at the end of a person's life or as hospice. More accurately, palliative care is a practice that focuses medical and caregivers' attention on improving a person's quality of life, as well as his or her length of survival. In other words, it seeks to prevent and relieve the suffering of persons living with serious illnesses, both during and after treatment.

One of the main goals of palliative care is to lessen the severity of symptoms caused by brain tumors, as well as the side effects from medical treatments. In this chapter, many common symptoms are addressed, along with methods to control them. As with any change in your health, make sure to track and share your symptoms with your medical team, paying close attention to how they may be changing over time.

In this chapter, you will learn the following:

- About the symptoms people with brain tumors commonly experience
- What palliative care means
- Which treatments help ease specific side effects
- Which "big picture" aspects of life are important to focus on now

Symptoms

Headache

Headache, a common symptom upon diagnosis, results from the pressure that develops from the growth of the brain tumor within the skull or on surrounding tissues. When this **intracranial pressure** (pressure exerted by the blood and brain volumes inside the skull) builds, headaches can be severe, particularly at night during sleep. Headaches can also occur after surgery, because of the surgical cuts and the moving of bone and muscle that occur during tumor removal. Common pharmaceutical treatments include dexamethasone, a strong steroid medication that decreases swelling; it is given in variable doses depending on the severity of the headache and associated swelling. Narcotics such as hydrocodone or oxycodone are also used or simple nonsteroidal anti-inflammatory drugs, such as ibuprofen two to four times daily.

Drop Attacks

When intracranial pressure remains elevated over a long period of time, a person may experience what is commonly known as a drop attack. This term describes the sudden loss of one's ability to stand. Typically, an individual's legs begin to shake before he or she drops to the floor fully conscious. Such episodes often occur after a long car ride or an extended amount of time spent sitting. They result from a sudden imbalance of blood pressure between the brain and the body. The best treatment is to avoid the situations that cause them or to slow down your movements. For instance, after a long period of sitting, carefully swing your legs to get the blood moving, take a few extra counts to stand up, or perhaps consider using a front-wheeled walker.

Seizures

When a growing tumor irritates the brain, abnormal electrical activity occurs, frequently resulting in a seizure. Simple seizures usually produce motor or sensory symptoms with no loss of consciousness. The type of seizure depends on the brain lobe involved. For instance, a tumor on the left side of the brain near the sensory strip will often cause a brief (1 to 2 minutes) episode of tingling or numbness in the right side of the body; similarly, a tumor in the motor strip of the right hemisphere might cause a simple rhythmic twitching of the face and hand of the left body. More complicated seizures may result in confusion or lack of awareness of the environment. For example, you might experience a simple seizure that spreads across the brain, causing a generalized tonic-clonic, or grand mal, seizure. A seizure of this type might produce rhythmic twitching or cause you to fall to the floor and perhaps lose bowel or bladder control. Seizures generally stop after a few minutes and may not require a trip to the emergency department. However, be sure to inform your treatment team about any seizure; your doctor may choose to change your seizure medications, often easily, over the telephone.

During and after surgery, seizure medications (or anticonvulsants) are typically prescribed to ease irritation or the electrical excitability of the brain to keep the person safe. This practice has been carefully reviewed in the medical literature. For persons who have never experienced a seizure, use of seizure medications beyond 1 month postsurgery is unlikely to be helpful. If seizures have occurred, however, the medications will need to be continued, often for at least a year and sometimes forever. Some seizure medications are known to lessen the efficacy of tumor treatments, namely chemotherapy. Because they are processed through the liver, such medications may reduce the effectiveness of chemotherapy by up to a quarter. As a result, older seizure medications, such as valproic acid, phenytoin, and carbamazepine, will generally need to be changed to levetiracetam or lamotrigine. Your medical team will prescribe the medications appropriate to your seizure pattern and condition.

For caregivers who observe a seizure episode, staying calm is the best first aid you can offer. The human body is smart and, if left alone, most seizures will stop on their own. Also, you might loosen a necktie and turn the head gently to one side to keep the airway clear. Contrary to popular wisdom, though, avoid placing anything into the person's mouth, as you could chip teeth or have a finger bitten! If three seizures occur in a row without the person waking up, this is a medical emergency called *status epilepticus*. Call 911 immediately and have the person transported to the closest hospital.

Nausea and Vomiting

Nausea and vomiting often result from high intracranial pressure or chemotherapy drugs. Such side effects are best remedied by taking oral chemotherapy in the evening with a large glass of water after a light meal, as well as regular doses of antinausea medications. Very strong antinausea medications include ondansetron (brand name Zofran) or dolasetron (Anzemet). On lower dose chemotherapy days, Phenergan taken orally or rectally is helpful, as are lorazepam and dexamethasone. Your doctor will work with you to identify the best combination of antinausea medications before the chemotherapy begins.

Constipation

With the use of oral temozolomide (Temodar), the most commonly prescribed chemotherapy drug for primary brain tumors, constipation is a common concern. To prevent it from becoming a serious issue, you will need to work in concert with your care providers to actively manage your diet, medication, and exercise routine. A diet containing plenty of fluids and fiber, including a lot of fresh fruits and vegetables, is important. During active chemotherapy days, two types of bowel medications offer relief: bisacodyl or another bulk-forming laxative acts as a stool softener, and senna encourages the bowel wall to contract, thereby improving regularity. Use of bisacodyl and senna together two to three times daily has proved beneficial in preventing constipation.

Deep Venous Thrombosis

Blood clots, also called deep venous thrombosis, that form in the calf and thigh often become problems for people with brain tumors. While they can occur in either leg, most often they form in the leg on the side of the body opposite to the brain tumor. Movement is an important way to prevent the development of blood clots. Regular walking or exercise that has you up on your feet and moving around will improve your circulation. You might also consider the use of compression stockings, which are effective in returning the blood supply and lymph to the heart; the downside is they are tight, difficult to put on, and many people find them impractical. A diet consisting of plenty of fluids is also valuable; keep a water bottle or teakettle at the ready. Warning signs of a possible blood clot include swelling and pain in the leg. If you experience these symptoms, make sure to bring it to the attention of your doctor, who will likely order an ultrasound study for confirmation. Treatments for blood clots include certain blood thinners, including enoxaparin or warfarin. Some doctors also may insert a small filter, shaped like a cocktail umbrella, in the large vein of the pelvis, which traps blood clots and keeps them from traveling to the lungs.

PCP Prophylaxis

Early in the course of treatment for brain tumors, radiation and daily chemotherapy are often taken together. During this phase, the white blood cell count will go down, leaving the person unprotected against infections. As a result, a type of pneumonia caused by *Pneumocystis jiroveci* (formerly called *Pneumocystis carinii* [PCP]), a fungus, can develop. This infection is very difficult to treat, so prevention is crucial. The recommended protocol is a double-strength antibiotic, sulfamethoxazole (Bactrim), taken three times a week. Once your white blood cell count returns to normal, and with your doctor's approval, you will likely be able to discontinue the antibiotic.

Fatigue

Chronic fatigue is a common symptom. It becomes especially noticeable in the middle of the radiation treatment cycle. Why radiation of the brain creates such fatigue is not well understood; nevertheless, it is very real and often quite predictable. Getting plenty of sleep, resting frequently during the day, taking naps, and avoiding work during radiation treatment are all good ways to minimize fatigue. Small doses of a stimulant such as methylphenidate (known commercially as Ritalin) can often be effective in increasing attentiveness, sharpening mental focus, and relieving fatigue and forgetfulness, foggy thinking, and other memory concerns. Also, after appropriate screening and evaluation, the use of antidepressants can be very helpful.

Changes in Taste

During radiation therapy of the brain, many patients have a metallic taste in their mouth or simply lose their appetite. This common problem is thought to be caused by damage to the rapidly dividing cells in the tongue as they come into contact with high doses of treatment. Dry mouth is another side effect should the salivary glands also be affected. A trip down the candy aisle may be your best option; lemon drops or other hard candy will mask the metallic taste. Also, frequent beverages and moist foods can be of help. Thankfully, this side effect tends to diminish over time. Still, it's important to continue to eat healthy foods to maintain your energy and avoid weight loss. Other strategies to try include increasing the salt content in food, experimenting with food consistency, and eating many small meals.

Cognitive Changes

Among the most vexing symptoms for people living with brain tumors are complications with memory and personality changes.

People with brain tumors can expect to experience a slowing of information processing and memory retrieval, and a reduced or lack of interest in activities that they used to enjoy. Because the frontal lobes are so large, they are the most common sites for brain tumor growth. When healthy, they function as the "executive" part of the brain, helping us wake up on time and get our tasks completed. Yet people with brain tumors sometimes get stuck on one task, repeating it over and over, or become easily distracted. Parties or other social settings may prove especially taxing; indeed, carrying on multiple conversations at the same time may become difficult and exhausting, even for the most outgoing of personalities. One way to reduce the strain is to get in the habit of making lists and attending more intimate social gatherings. Also, medications used in the management of dementia (disorders of thinking and memory) might prove helpful.

Aphasia

Aphasia describes a difficulty with language, often resulting from left temporal-parietal lobe tumors within the speech center. With aphasia, a person knows what she or he wants to say but cannot say it, has trouble understanding what is being said by others, or both. Nouns and the names of things can be especially difficult to access. Anyone with a language difficulty of any kind will benefit from an evaluation by a speech and language therapist. Your specific challenges can be reviewed and strategies for working around them can be developed. One possibility is to communicate more frequently through the use of pictures and/or a letter board.

Visual Field Deficits

Occipital lobe tumors may make it difficult to see to the left or right side. This is a problem for reading, cycling, and other sports, and, above all, for driving. With visual difficulties to the left in particular, the person is not always aware of the problem, which could lead to falls or accidents. You will want to have a frank conversation with your doctor about your transit needs and ongoing ability to drive safely.

Reading

The vision field problems mentioned earlier, combined with aphasia, can make reading difficult. Perhaps you are experiencing this difficulty right now as you scan this chapter. You might try using a ruler to keep your eye moving along the line or choosing large-print books, which are available at many public libraries. Books on tape or CDs or podcasts are also excellent substitutes.

Hemiparesis

Hemiparesis describes weakness, or partial paralysis, that affects an arm, leg, or both on the same side of the body. Often stiff and painful, the weakened limb is likely to benefit from physical therapy, while medications such as baclofen and diazepam will help loosen it up as well. Visits with a rehabilitation physician (also known as a physiatrist) might also be helpful. For weakness of the foot, a lightweight plastic ankle brace with an adjustable strap around the knee (called an ankle-foot-orthosis [AFO]) will keep the foot up, preventing you from stumbling.

Depression

Depression can certainly accompany a cancer diagnosis, but it is not as common as you might think. To the outside observer, the cognitive changes described earlier often resemble clinical depression; indeed, it can be difficult to distinguish one from the other, as both depression and cognitive changes frequently occur together.

You and your caregiver know your moods and temperament best, so it is vital to share with your medical team any changes in your daily behaviors, thinking, eating, or sleeping patterns. In confirmed cases of depression, antidepressant medications will be prescribed. Sometimes formal neuropsychological testing, performed under the direction of a psychologist, is needed to understand mood issues.

Steroid Myopathy

A myopathy is a weakening of the skeletal muscle, in this case related to excessive corticosteroid levels in the body caused by the use of a steroid to reduce brain swelling. Dexamethasone, a commonly used steroid, is most frequently prescribed at the lowest effective dose, which ranges from 0.5 mg twice daily to 8 mg four times daily. This is the "holy water" of brain tumor treatment. Swelling of the brain around a tumor is a significant problem; such swelling creates a great deal of pressure within the hard, unyielding skull. Dexamethasone shrinks the swelling, or excess water, that collects around most tumors, thereby relieving any headache, weakness, or other neurologic problems that commonly develop. Over time, its side effects will increase, although they vary in severity from person to person. Common side effects include bone loss, high blood sugars, agitation or mood changes, leg swelling, insomnia, and weakness of the hip muscles, which makes rising from a low chair difficult. Regular exercise of the hip girdle muscles by, for instance, riding a stationary bicycle will prevent some muscle weakness, as will a gradual tapering off of the medication. *Gradual* is an important word here—the medication, when stopped suddenly, produces severe joint pain in elbows, hips, and knees. Again, individual responses differ; some people can taper off steroid medications quickly, while others remain steroid dependant.

Rash

Many patients experience an itchy, bumpy rash that spreads quickly over the trunk, front, and back, and often includes the arms and legs. It is most likely caused by the seizure medications phenytoin, lamotrigine, or levetiracetam. Itching can be treated with diphenhydramine (known over the counter as Benadryl) and topical steroid creams. The rash tends to goes away when the seizure medication is stopped or replaced with another type.

"Big Picture" Topics to Keep in Mind

> "Get over the fear of being able to talk about things. You're not going to make anyone die sooner."
> —Nancy, whose husband, Randy, died of cerebellar medulloblastoma in 2006.

The following quality-of-life issues are also important, because they contribute to an individual's sense of self, identity, independence, interactions with others, and place in the world. Feel free to keep them in mind and, at the level of your comfort, to talk about them with your medical team and your loved ones.

Sexuality

A cancer diagnosis does not necessarily diminish the desire for sexual intimacy. Indeed, the physical and emotional connection made through sexual contact can have a profoundly restorative effect on an individual's or couple's sense of normalcy and well-being. If fatigue or depression makes sexual activity more challenging or less pleasurable, then masturbation, mutual caressing, and physical closeness remain wonderful options. Make it clear to your medical team the value you place on your sexuality and any limitations or frustrations you may be experiencing. Your doctor can offer medications, such as sildenafil (Viagra) or tadalafil (Cialis), to help with erectile dysfunction, and over-the-counter lubricants are readily available to counter vaginal dryness. If seizure medications have dampened your interest in sex, your care team can prescribe other options. For those in a committed relationship, it is also important to have a conversation with your partner about each of your feelings related to your illness.

Spirituality

Spirituality means many things to many people. It may mean for you a resounding faith in the tenets of organized religion and the sense of community that instills. Or it may describe a belief in the earth's numerous wonders, a quest for a cosmic foothold in the world, or a search for purpose in life. Spirituality, especially when connected to an organized religion, can offer patients a ready-made community of people ready to give support—from food to transportation to emotional support and prayers. It may also offer answers to some big questions you may be grappling with right now. No matter the nature of your spiritual orientation, each of us has interests in life that make us unique and important and that we can draw from in this challenging time. Talk to your doctors about your short-term and long-term goals to make sure your treatment approach fits into your spiritual life.

Dick, who was diagnosed with a glioblastoma multiforme in 2004, was placed on hospice 3 years later. Contrary to what many people imagine, he remembers the experience as "lots of fun" and was sorry to see the hospice workers go once his cancer went into remission. "These are interesting people," he says. "They drop in on you,

and they're full of laughter. [But] as soon as they found out I was not
fatal, they stopped coming. That's one of their rules. When it was
over, it was over."

Hospice

It is often said that hospice is not about *dying*, but about *living* every
day as fully as possible. Still, many people understandably fear hospice because they believe it means that active medical treatment of
the brain tumor has stopped. For many, this is true. The option of
hospice is often raised when the restorative possibilities of remaining treatments are outweighed by their negative side effects and
when the care team believes that an individual has 6 months or
fewer to live. Yet hospice can be a remarkable time, for both patient
and caregiver. It can lift the daily responsibilities off the shoulders
of the caregiver, freeing up valuable time to spend with family,
friends, and one on one, while offering compassionate support and
counseling by trained professionals right in the home.

Supervised by your primary medical caregiver, the hospice
experience is designed to keep your care centered at home instead
of at the clinic. Some communities offer inpatient hospice facilities, but these are somewhat uncommon. At the outset, you will
be visited at home by a social worker, a nurse, and occupational
and physical therapists, who set up home visits depending on your
needs. They will also try to anticipate and alleviate any problems
you might have, such as from constipation, pain, or fatigue.

> "Make sure people live up to the moment they don't live."
> —Nancy , whose efforts to back a Death with Dignity
> initiative resulted in a Washington state law that allows ter-
> minally ill patients to end their lives, in tribute to her late
> husband, Randy.

Death and Dying

How does a person with a brain tumor die? Thankfully, with very little pain and a slow drifting off to sleep. As a tumor grows, the pressure inside the brain and skull begins to rise. The result is an increasing sleepiness. Gradually, over days to weeks, the person spends less time awake and more time asleep. Once he or she stops waking up, a coma sets in. Without food or water, the patient will drift away and die of dehydration within about 10 days. This last period of time can be hard on loved ones, although the person is unaware of what is happening. Throughout the dying process, the person will continue to need compassionate tending. The hospice team will come frequently at this point and is available 24 hours a day to give practical advice and psychological support. Any new symptoms are dealt with quickly by hospice calls to the doctor. This way the person and his or her loved ones can enjoy their time together unencumbered with managing medical care. Bodily functions, such as urination and defection, can be handled using a diaper or a bladder catheter. To avoid bedsores, muscles can be massaged and the person's torso and limbs can be turned frequently, and gently, in bed. A dry mouth can be moistened with a sponge.

Those who are dying do not usually feel much hunger, but small amounts of food can be given for texture or comfort. When the person is in a coma, any steroid medication used to control the increased pressure can be discontinued, and other medications to control seizures may need to be given in a different way. The use of artificial means to extend life, such as intravenous fluids and feeding tubes, is not recommended now, as it would only prolong suffering.

Chapter 6

Care of the Caregiver

"God bless the caregivers, because they really have a tough job,"
says Christopher, who has lived with an oligodendroglioma
for 11 years. His wife has seen her responsibilities grow while
Christopher, the father of two teens, left his blue-collar job and
took on a "Mr. Mom" homemaker role. "She has to deal with my
disease, her career, and the kids. To watch your spouse decline,
that's rough."

Caregivers are central to a patient's medical treatment, daily care, and—in most instances—quality of life. A primary caregiver may be a spouse, a parent, a sibling, or even a close friend. No matter the relationship, the caregiver is an individual who is deeply invested in helping the patient cope with the diagnosis and treatment. Oftentimes the caregiver's role is complex and performed while holding down a job. That role may also include becoming a medical expert, advocating for the patient's care, coordinating appointments and schedules, maintaining the household, paying the bills, keeping the kids fed, the dogs walked, the cats off the kitchen table, and so on.

A daunting role, to be sure, being a caregiver requires compassion, fortitude, and a fierce resilience. It means watching your loved one weather difficult surgery, treatments, and personality changes. It means being a cheerleader when hope feels scarce and managing one's own emotional ups and downs through the process, which can span months or years.

Caregivers are also just people, not saints or superheroes. If you are a caregiver who's feeling fear, uncertainty, denial, hope, anger, shock, or numb, you're nothing but normal. Every patient, every tumor, every treatment is unique. Nonetheless, some similarities exist. This section will offer some general suggestions to guide caregivers toward a better experience for everyone involved.

In this chapter, you will learn the following:

- **What you need to know now—and in the months to come**
- **Ways to streamline communications with family and friends**
- **Tips for preparing for appointments**
- **Tips for reorganizing your household**
- **How treatment is likely to change your loved one**
- **The importance of taking care of yourself**

"Resilience comes from the willingness to ask for help, to say what help you need and what you don't need, and to adapt as the situation changes," says Nancy, whose husband, Randy, died of cerebellar medulloblastoma in 2006. Nancy started a brain tumor support group for caregivers and became the "poster child" of Washington State's Death with Dignity initiative, which became law in 2009. She also is the source of much of the wisdom contained in this chapter.

"My husband never regretted getting that brain cancer," Nancy says. "It taught him to love harder than he ever would have."

Presurgery

Secure Your Oxygen Mask

A tip from the airline industry is, "Secure your oxygen mask over your nose and mouth before assisting others." In other words, to help people, you must first take care of yourself. As a caregiver, you may not be sleeping well, your routines may be off, and your mood may not be the best. Check in with your own doctor and, perhaps, a counselor to monitor your health and well-being. Find ways to laugh and to indulge your pleasures. These will boost your physical and emotional energy to support the patient.

Be Willing to Help Direct the Medical Decisions

It's for the patient to decide the quality and quantity of life he or she wants. Patients will respond better—to surgery, to treatments, to you—if they choose their approach and are empowered to make their own decisions. If the patient is too young or is unable to make choices independently, then you will need to weigh in. If surgery is proposed, help the patient stay in the moment and focus on getting through the operation.

Put Your Affairs in Order

If you have not already done so, this is a good prompt to prepare wills, medical directives, powers of attorney, and to prearrange funeral or memorial services for both of you. Although such arrangements are difficult to confront, many people describe a feeling of relief and reassurance once they have taken care of these things. It is especially important when you confront a serious illness. Review your medical insurance policy. Surgery and treatment are very expensive. If you don't have adequate assets or sufficient medical coverage, look into options under Social Security, Medicare, or Medicaid. The decisions you make—or don't make—now may affect your financial options later.

Ask Questions, Gather Information

Information is a powerful tool. Ask questions of your doctors and of your medical team, and take notes. Keep a list of new questions as they arise. Seek out written information, and re-read it periodically throughout the process because what may not make sense today may be useful to you in the months to come. Start keeping a journal. This will be an important source of historical information over time.

Fortify Your Communication Network

Pick one person to serve as your primary contact for family and friends during the hospital stay and recuperation. Relay information to that person to avoid getting bogged down in repeated calls of concern. Group e-mails are another good tool, as are online options, such as CaringBridge.com, a service that lets you post updates and photographs. This is a good time to obtain an e-mail address or to get a cell phone if you do not already have them.

> After Pamela's emergency surgery to biopsy two glioblastoma multiforme tumors, the home phone started ringing off the hook. Her husband, Charlie, initially fought the idea of employing online communications tools, but he soon relented. CaringBridge, he says, "saved my life." Charlie learned to answer calls from concerned friends and family this way: "Go to CaringBridge, read that, then call me tomorrow," he says. "In one fell swoop, they're up to speed."

Arrange a Signal

Consider having a preplanned, nonverbal sign to let the patient know you are there while he or she is in the hospital recovering from surgery. It may be a kiss on the hand or a gentle stroke on the cheek. Talk about it before surgery. Whatever you decide, make it something comforting that helps the patient feel loved and involves minimal sensory stimulation.

Plan Fun

Together, plan something to look forward to postsurgery and throughout the treatment period that indulges both of you. It may be a short daytrip to a special destination or a meal at a favorite restaurant. It may be a fun gift or a massage. If you have a special friend, relative, or child, plan to spend time with that person. Attaching something pleasurable to a stressful time will help create balance in your life so that the brain tumor isn't your sole focus.

During Treatment

What Can We Do Now?

It's natural for us to want to know why something has happened. But much is still unknown about the causes of brain cancer. Asking why is not helpful to the patient, the caregiver, or the family. What does help is asking, "What are we going to do about it now?" Such forward-looking questions help the patient focus on choices to consider and future plans to make.

Laugh, Cry, Be Real

The stark truth is that treating brain tumors is often more about increasing the length of life relatively free of neurologic symptoms than curing the cancer. You can either laugh or cry at the situation, and sometimes you'll need to do both. Tears of laughter are a medicine that you should incorporate into this journey. Watch a favorite movie together. Read jokes to each other. Try as hard as you can to approach these changes with humor and grace versus sadness and hopelessness.

Join a Support Group

We all need camaraderie and support. Try to find a support group for those living with a brain cancer patient. The experiences of such caregivers are very different from those living with someone who has a disease affecting another organ or body part. Whether in person or online, a support group offers valuable opportunities to swap stories, challenges, frustrations, solutions, and important resources, and it can help you deal with all the changes in your life.

Help the Patient Decide When or Whether to Return to Work

Each patient's course is different, and there's no one right answer. Many people with benign tumors are able to work while undergoing treatment, and they may relish the stability of their work routines. Others, however, will opt for taking a short-term medical leave while focusing their energies on recovery. In the case of malignant tumors, most individuals choose to take extended time off of work—though, again, not all. Surgery and treatment (if necessary) will damage the brain in ways that might affect work performance. Although your loved one may feel well following surgery, delayed side effects, both physical and mental, may occur weeks or months after surgery. To recover, the brain will need all its strength, without the additional stress created by work. Unquestionably a difficult financial—and, in our workaholic culture, personal—decision, not working can be a rare gift to be enjoyed as the patient gathers strength and recuperates. What's more, a patient's return to work may affect his or her eligibility for disability insurance, which may be needed should side effects develop.

Weigh Options

When deciding on the best strategy for treatment, the person with a brain tumor will need to decide on not only the type of treatment but also who will provide it. It is also important to take into consideration the effects those treatments will have on the person with the tumor (and, thus, on you). You may want to look for a neuro-oncologist near your home. While undergoing treatment a long distance away may assure patients that they are receiving the "best" care, it may tax them, you, and others in your care team. Today, information—X-rays, lab tests, treatment options, and so on—can be shared electronically between doctors so that excellent care may not require you to travel far.

At the same time, a multidisciplinary neuro-oncology program can add a lot to the care of your loved one. Neuro-oncologists are able to evaluate neurologic examinations, read magnetic resonance imaging (MRI) scans, treat neurologic symptoms such as seizures, as well as provide chemotherapy as treatment for the tumor. Multidisciplinary neuro-oncology programs are usually located in large population centers. If there is not a neuro-oncologist near your home, you may be able to assemble a team locally of your primary care provider and a medical oncologist who can work together with your neuro-oncologist at a distance. Often patients choose to have the 6-week intensive daily radiation treatments in their own communities but then travel once a month to once every 3 months to see their neuro-oncologist for continuity of care. Help the person with the tumor to weigh options, but support his or her decision.

Attend Appointments

Some weeks will be filled with appointments. Attend as many of these appointments as you can, or find someone who can go in your place. Bring paper and a pen, and be prepared to ask questions, in addition to providing a summary of the events that have taken place since the last visit. Stress ransacks memory, so expect to forget some of what is communicated; your notes will be your backup memory. Expect the doctor to present information in an honest and kind manner and to take time to answer your questions. In turn, air your concerns and observations about symptoms and side effects the person with the tumor is experiencing.

Become an Advocate

Becoming an advocate means promoting the wishes of your loved one—and also, perhaps, guarding against anyone, whether a doctor, family member, or friend, who does not support those wishes. In this role, you may need to learn to say no to those who tell the patient what he or she should do, think, or believe. Let those individuals know that what will be helpful is for them to support whatever the patient chooses. Should your loved one's ability to make decisions about his or her care diminish, your role as advocate will become more important than ever.

Embrace Change

Becoming a caregiver means seeing your own role evolve, often in dramatic ways. The power dynamic may shift, responsibilities may be reassigned, and long-established patterns in your relationship may fade. Be open to the possibility that some of these changes may be positive ones.

> *Salli, whose husband, John, was diagnosed with cerebellar astrocytoma, wishes her family could put brain cancer behind it. "I would love for this to be over," she says. Nevertheless, given a choice of having brain cancer enter her life or not, she vows she would choose it. "A lot of good has come out of this," she says.*

For instance, John, whose work often kept him away from home and family, has since discovered new interests and priorities, and his family relationships have grown extremely close. Also, before John's tumor, Salli called herself "one of those wives who just loved having my husband do everything. I didn't even drive in downtown Seattle; I didn't like traffic." Now, she's the family's breadwinner and commutes with confidence. "The first time, I was white-knuckled," she says. "Now it's nothing. I've become more independent and stronger."

Remember That Each Individual Is Unique

Doctors formulate a prognosis and treatment plan based on their experience. But remember: each person is unique. How he or she responds to treatments and side effects depends on many factors, not least of which include genetics, strength, personality, and individual spirit. Statistics and prediction charts are tools physicians use to assess overall prognosis. They allow a frank discussion of what you can practically expect in the future.

Expect Side Effects from the Cancer-Fighting Treatment

Treatments—surgery, radiation, chemotherapy—affect healthy cells along with the cancerous ones. According to some patients and caregivers, the effects of treatments can be worse than the brain tumor itself. Side effects may include extreme fatigue, hair and eyelash loss, changes in sight and hearing, loss of balance, changes in speech, seizures, disorientation, aggression, depression, dietary intolerances, nausea and vomiting, loss of short-term memory, and changes in personality. Update your medical team at every visit regarding potential side effects.

Expect Symptoms from the Brain Tumor

What's unique about brain cancer is that whatever your loved one is experiencing today can change just as quickly tomorrow. Some symptoms can be profound and sudden while others may be subtle and observed only through daily living together. Ask the doctor how you should communicate such changes to the medical staff. Some symptoms can be minimized through physical therapy, counseling, medications, or good health practices, such as rest and light exercise. Also, some side effects will inform the doctor about how the patient is responding to treatment or how the cancer is progressing.

"Brain cancer changes who a person is at their core," says caregiver Nancy. "It changes their personality, who they are. Your treatment is attacking the part of your body that affects everything about you." What's more, the symptoms from the tumor can often cause cognitive and behavioral shifts.

In her husband's unique case, she noted three interesting changes: Randy tapped a creative outlet—making bookmarks for the elementary students he read to; he never passed up an opportunity to tell a loved one he loved them; and he developed an obsession for three gold pens. "He'd get very agitated without those pens in his hand," she says.

Identify Your Core Team

People want to help. Some will prove helpful, and others will not. You might be surprised by who rises like cream to the top. Such supporters may be in your immediate family, from your family of friends, or among your acquaintances. They may be your co-workers, your former teachers, or the neighborhood kid down the block. Your cast of supporters may change over time, so be open to that fluidity. Offer them ongoing assignments, or ask when they'd like to help out and how.

Create Your A, B, and C Teams

Team A consists of people who are handy in crisis mode, take direction, don't offer their opinions unless asked, and can deal with medical situations, including blood and other bodily fluids. These are your firefighters. You can count on them for everything from responding to an emergency, to gathering detailed information at doctor appointments, to watching videos at the homestead while you do something nice for yourself.

Team B is made up of good maintenance people. They can pick up your groceries, mow your lawn, and take your kids out. They won't necessarily help the patient, but they'll give you more time to spend with him or her.

Team C consists of people you may love but who cannot handle the stress, responsibility, or vulnerability that comes with living with cancer. They may not support, and may even undermine, the patient's wishes, and they may create unnecessary drama and distractions. Unfortunately, such people can be close relatives or good friends. To harness all your resources in support of the patient, you may choose to distance yourself or disconnect from them, if only for now.

Accept People's Limitations

Good, caring people sometimes have trouble knowing what to say in the face of illness. Team C, for instance, may be afraid of saying the wrong thing. It doesn't mean they don't care; they simply may not know what to say or fear saying the wrong thing.

You may find yourself needing to reassure others, letting them know that sometimes just a hand squeeze will do, or that simple conversation about the normal stuff of daily life is important to you now.

> *"Not long after Adrienne was diagnosed, she went to a reception,"* says Simeon Rubenstein, MD, *of his wife of 42 years, who is living with a high-grade astrocytoma of the thalamus (a structure deep inside the brain). "About a third of the people came up to her and said, 'We heard, we're sorry.' A third acknowledged her, and about a third ignored her." "I'm convinced that each group is concerned about Adrienne,"* he says. *"It has more to do about comfort level than concern. I would say, 'Don't be afraid to say hi.' You don't need to talk about cancer. You just need to show your friendship."*

Arrange Transportation

On days you need a break, set up a schedule for your A and B teams to drive the patient to and from appointments. Don't try to do this alone. They want to help, and you need the help; it's a good match.

Prepare Your Home

During treatment, the person with the tumor may feel sick. Have a variety of foods and drinks on hand, as an interest in nourishment can change dramatically from day to day. Treatment can affect how she or he tastes food; favorites may not taste good now. Encourage your loved one to eat or drink whatever and however much he or she can tolerate.

Read Prescriptions

Radiation, chemotherapy, and prescription medications all cause side effects. Read the literature that comes with any prescription or treatment. Keep it nearby to refer to should a side effect occur later. Do not expect the doctor to know all the side effects of every treatment and every medication. A trusted pharmacist can be very helpful.

Create Rituals

For instance, if your loved one's hair is likely to fall out, create a ritual or celebration around shaving his or her head to embrace, and destigmatize, the new cue-ball look. Some family members might even join in. And periodic gifts of scarves and hats can also perk up the patient's look and outlook. For individuals with short-term memory loss, use colored sticky notes around the house. For balance problems, consider a nice walking stick instead of a cane; you can find one at a sporting goods store or have one carved for you. Give nicknames to the new physical aides to reflect the patient's personality, not the medical condition.

Stay Active

Exercising will help relieve the physical and mental stress both of you are experiencing. Encourage your loved one to stay as active as possible, such as doing chores around the house. Don't give up your daily dog walks, swimming laps, mountain bike rides, or whatever makes you feel your best. Make sure you continue to find pleasure and laughter in your life.

Accept New Limits

Over time, patients with brain tumors may develop different limitations. Cognitive abilities that involve higher level thinking, such as planning and financial decision making, may be affected. Recognition of loved ones, events, or places could diminish. This loss can affect their ability to care for children, to drive a car, or to handle other situations that require quick decisions. It may be helpful to make a scrapbook of pictures with references to loved ones and meaningful events. You may find that local car or grocery delivery services can be helpful. Whatever the need may be, acknowledge this change, and make necessary adjustments. Your local cancer center or the patient's doctor's office may have a listing of available community resources.

Develop New Routines

Keep a calendar that reminds the patient of the day's activities. Review information in a loving manner. If the patient is able, encourage him or her to keep up with housework, lawn care, or whatever feels useful.

> "I do all the meal planning and cooking," says Christopher, a tumor patient. "I take care of the house. I'm Mr. Mom. I'd go crazy without it."

Encourage Rest

Your loved one's ability to respond to new information, instructions, and verbal cues may slow down. His or her openness to deal with sensory stimuli (sounds, sight, touch, taste, smell) may not be what it once was. Social functions can be especially tiring. Remind family and friends that it takes a lot of energy to be around others. Sufficient down time each day to rest the patient's brain will help, especially before a social event.

Provide Emergency Information

A person whose brain is damaged from cancer may not be as obviously impaired as someone who has lost a limb. But his or her impairment is no less significant. Place a card in the patient's wallet or pocket that contains your primary doctor's phone number, medications being taken, and your emergency number.

Limit Stimuli

The person with a brain tumor may do better in a quieter, less distracting environment. Try to limit how much the TV is left on as a companion or distraction. Keep life simple and enjoyable. Select entertainment that's at a slower pace, such as reading aloud and soft music.

Help the Patient Find Fun and Meaning

After treatment has ended, if the patient chooses not to return to work, help him or her find something meaningful to engage in. Volunteering at a local grade school, retirement home, or food bank can be immensely rewarding for patients. It helps them interact with people and develop new interests while making a contribution to society.

> *John volunteers at a nearby assisted living center, which he reaches by bus. "I like being around people who aren't so worried about me," he says. "They just want to have fun." During his twice-weekly visits, they play a horseracing game John built. Asked whether the residents were gambling, he exclaims, "YES, big time! They tell me if I'm not there, it's not as fun."*

Salli, John's wife, beams over reports of John's activities. "I've been with him to the retirement center, and I have to say, I was more proud of him there," she says, "than at his former job. Not only did he ride the bus, but he taught the people at the retirement center how to ride the bus." For his work, John was named Commuter of the Year. "He turned into a hero," she says.

Recurrence

Discuss Options

Should the cancer recur, you and the person with a brain tumor need to have another straightforward discussion with the neuro-oncologist about life expectancy with or without additional treatment. Trust one another and have an honest and sensitive discussion on the patient's desired outcome and what is realistic. If the side effects from treatment have been well tolerated up until now, continued treatment may be reasonable. If treatment will reduce quality of life, taking away valuable time with no increased life expectancy, then the patient should carefully consider how he or she wants to spend the time remaining. This is an excellent time to explore hospice options and to understand what additional help can be provided. The Medicare hospice benefit allows for increased care in the home by hospice nurses, social workers, and physical therapists and can be utilized if there is some possibility that survival might be as short as 6 months. Generally, patients and their families make a decision that they want to forgo additional treatments aimed at treating the tumor for treatments that focus more on palliation of symptoms and focus on everyday quality of life.

Clarify the Patient's Goals

Each patient, each tumor, is different. In most cases concerning benign tumors, the immediate goal will likely be to get beyond the treatment course and return to daily life, with intermittent check-ins with your medical team. However, in the case of individuals with malignant tumors, it's important to have a heart-to-heart about how your loved one envisions living the rest of his or her life. Encourage the patient to communicate those goals to the doctor. You may need to take a more active role in these discussions if he or she has diminished memory and cognitive skills. You will need to help the patient understand the options and the expected results. Keep in mind that the doctor's goal is to treat the patient, but that your loved one's goal is incorporating treatment into his or her life.

Accept Your Loved One's Wishes

Many people rely on the doctor to make the decision of when treatment should end. But it is not the doctor's choice; it's the patient's choice. Your loved one may choose to restart treatment. Or he or she may choose to live life free of doctor's appointments and treatment. But it is the patient's choice, which you must accept, support, and embrace. Make sure the patient isn't continuing treatment because of your fears about death.

> Hospice "was marvelous support for me," says Nancy, whose husband, Dick, was diagnosed with a glioblastoma multiforme tumor in 2004. The Clevelands had hospice workers come to their home to help with Dick's care and to do the "cruddy stuff," Nancy says. "They are fabulous people, and they are there for you," Nancy says. "They really relieve you and take your burden away so you can deal with the person you love."

Consider Hospice

Be willing to ask the doctor whether it's time for hospice. Hospice care helps you both through the next stage. It provides resources for physical, emotional, and financial needs that make the last part of an individual's life meaningful and profoundly loving. It can bring a strong sense of relief, as patients receive care at a specialized level, freeing you up to enjoy your time together. Let the patient know that if the situation improves, hospice will leave. If you and the patient are uncomfortable discussing it, ask a social worker or religious leader to assist you. And remind family and friends that the patient is still very much alive.

Prepare for Death

All of us will die. Intellectually, we know that, but in our hearts we don't want to accept it. The patient has the benefit that most of us do not: knowing in advance that he or she is likely to die in the near future. This knowledge gives the patient continued control over options he or she has about how to spend the remainder of time left. This time gives you both the opportunity to say the things that should be said. And remember: Your loved one will not die any sooner by discussing his or her choices.

Help Your Loved One Plan His or Her Memorial Service

Propose that the patient be involved in the planning of his or her memorial service or funeral. What type of service does he or she want? Who will officiate or speak? Where should the ceremony take place? How elaborate or how simple? What should the obituary say? Which music should be played? How would the patient like to be remembered? A grave marker? A tree planted? Would the patient like to donate any organs to research? Let the patient guide these discussions, with the help of trained hospice staff.

Indulge in Life's Pleasures

Now is a time for your loved one to eat, drink, and do whatever it is that makes him or her feel good, so long as it's safe for all involved. Indulge yourselves with a massage and manicure-pedicure, a harpist who makes house calls, ice cream for breakfast, chocolate in bed, a new haircut, humorous movies—whatever will make you both feel pampered. Find laughter and joy amid the difficulties. As Nancy says, "When you've got limited time, and if you know what's going to kill you, you can really have fun."

> After electing not to pursue further treatment for two aggressive glioblastoma multiforme tumors, Pam announced a new staple for cocktail hour: "I'm only having Veuve Clicquot champagne!" Her husband, Charlie, was happy to oblige, noting that they were probably the only residents of San Juan Island to buy the swanky bubbly "by the six-pack."

Share the Love

Many of us would like to be at our own memorial service, hearing what people say about us. We listen to eulogies after our loved ones' deaths; why not before they die? With the patient's approval, ask family and friends to write what the patient means to them and, if they wish, to read it to him or her. This can be very comforting and rewarding for a patient to hear. Encourage family and friends to tell one another how they feel, to share stories, and to laugh and reminisce with the patient.

Heal Each Other

Reflect on your life together. Reminisce. Invite your core support-ers to share in this time. Give yourself breaks to keep up your own emotional and physical strength. Continue to care for yourself. Look for laughter. Love your loved one and accept love in return. Enjoy the time you have together.

Chapter 7

Planning for Your Future

Managing Your Personal Affairs

Murray Sagsveen, JD, and Laurie Hanson, JD

We all know in theory that we should plan for unexpected family emergencies, such as the diagnosis of a chronic illness. Day-to-day matters often allow us to push this kind of planning to the bottom of our "to do" list, however. Planning for emergencies by necessity involves difficult family discussions that we might prefer to avoid. However, addressing difficult family decisions before an emergency arises is usually far easier than coping with them during an emergency.

To illustrate, consider the following example:

John visited his aging mother, Bertha, and they discussed the importance of an advance directive and a power of attorney. Bertha insisted that she did not want the family to take any unusual life-prolonging measures if something were to happen so that she could not make decisions for herself. She asked that John handle her finances if she were to become unable to do so. After this conversation, John made an appointment with his mother's attorney, and after several more discussions among the three of them, Bertha decided to sign an advance directive and a durable power of attorney. A month later, Bertha had a severe stroke that did in fact leave her unable to communicate.

If John had not started this discussion with his mother about an advance directive and power of attorney, Bertha's other children might never have learned about her end-of-life wishes. Had John and Bertha not taken the time to have an advance directive and power of attorney discussed, drafted, and signed, John would not have been able to handle even routine financial matters for his mother after her stroke.

This chapter explains the importance of planning for the future *and* provides useful information to assist you and your family with these details. You will learn ways to ensure that your affairs are managed as you want them to be managed— even if you are no longer able to communicate or make decisions yourself.

You will learn about the following:

- **Informal arrangements with friends or family**
- **Formal arrangements with or without court involvement**
  - **To manage your financial affairs such as powers of attorney, trusts, and conservatorships**
  - **To manage your health care through health care directives, living wills, POLST, DNR/DNI/DNHs, or guardianships**
- **To ensure that your post-death wishes are followed regarding your property and the disposition of your body**

Your Emergency Notebook

A first step in planning for emergencies is assembling and maintaining key health, financial, and other information in one place so that family members and caregivers may access the information if you are suddenly unable to communicate with them. Many organizations have developed planning guides that are free for members. But you can also create your own "emergency notebook" with a three-ring binder and a set of divider tabs. Organize your emergency notebook as follows, with tabs for separating documents into the following sections:

1. Emergency contact information
   - Spouse, partner, or significant other
   - Children
   - Siblings
   - Parents
2. Financial and legal contact information
   - Estate attorney
   - Accountant
   - Investment advisor
3. Medical information
   - Medication (recent, past, and present)
   - Contact information for both primary care and specialist physicians
   - Immunization records
   - Significant medical, dental, and eye care details (including the physicians' names and locations of medical records)
   - Allergies
   - Significant family medical history
4. Financial information
   - Bank accounts
   - Insurance policies
   - Retirement plans
   - Stocks and bonds
   - Recurring bills (for example: utilities, insurance, mortgage payments)

- Real and personal property
- Loans (receivable and payable)
- Financial powers of attorney
- Taxes (location of past tax returns and information for current tax year)
- Safe deposit box

5. End-of-life information
   - Will and any accompanying statement concerning final arrangements for personal property
   - Advance directive
   - Organ donor information
   - Funeral and burial guidance

6. Location of key items
   - Important documents (for example: passports, military records, deeds, marriage license, Social Security numbers, titles to vehicles)
   - Photos
   - Jewelry

7. Passwords and electronic media (Passwords are vital, and given that they frequently change, don't forget to update your emergency notebook, even if by hand.)
   - Home and office computers
   - Software programs
   - Financial and medical Web sites
   - Facebook and similar pages (consider, for instance, how you want these handled after your death)

Of course, an emergency notebook is not helpful if family members cannot find or access it. When discussing the contents of your emergency notebook with family members, be sure to explain where the notebook is located.

Informal and Formal Arrangements

A second step in emergency planning is to make arrangements for events that may be anticipated or unanticipated. Depending on the circumstance, the arrangements made will be either informal or formal.

Informal Care Arrangements

Informal arrangements are temporary and can usually be made with family, friends, and neighbors. For example, if you have surgery scheduled and know that you will be unable to perform normal household chores while you are recuperating (an anticipated event), you may want to line up family members or friends to assist with your medication, grocery shopping, cooking, transportation to medical appointments, or housekeeping. You may also want them to help with financial matters, such as writing out checks, filling out tax returns, and balancing the checkbook. Such informal arrangements are very common and, in fact, make up the majority of assistance to people who are temporarily or permanently living with disabilities.

Entrusting private financial or medical information to family members or friends, however, may have unintended negative consequences. It may result in uncomfortable situations that may even have financially or medically harmful consequences. In such cases, formal arrangements are preferable. Formal arrangements may include legal safeguards regarding supervision and record-keeping, or review by an outside party to minimize the risk of exploitation by an informal caregiver. Similarly, formal arrangements may also be made to protect the caregiver, who may later be questioned regarding legitimate reimbursement for services.

Even when informal arrangements work well, the day may come when more formal arrangements are needed.

Formal Financial Management Services

When planning for the future, it is important to know what financial management services are available for your individual needs. These services are listed next, starting from the least to the most formal.

Automatic Banking and Direct Deposit

Modern banking technology, such as automatic bill payment and direct deposit, can help you with your finances. At a minimum, Social Security payments and pension income should be set up so they are directly deposited. Utilities and insurance payments should also be set up to be withdrawn automatically from your account. Doing so can prevent you from unintentionally discontinuing your health insurance or from having your electricity shut off. It is wise to have one "working" bank account, such as a checking account, into which income is deposited and from which monthly bills are paid.

To arrange for Social Security checks to be deposited directly to a bank account, you may call Social Security at 1–800–772–1213 and ask for a direct deposit form or sign up on the Social Security Direct Deposit page online at http://www.ssa.gov/deposit/. A bank can also provide you with this form. Beginning in 2013, all Social Security recipients will be required to have checks directly deposited.

Multiple-Name Bank Accounts

Adding a name to a bank account is an easy and effective way to allow a trusted relative or friend to provide informal help. By having access to the account, that person can help sign checks, pay bills, or transfer money between your accounts. That person can also have access to bank records to monitor electronic deposits, ensure that all bills are paid on time, and review monthly statements to ensure that nothing is amiss in all your accounts.

Several types of multiple-name bank accounts are available, each with different rules. Any type of account—for example, savings, checking, and certificates of deposit—may be held in more than one name. Such accounts are easy to set up just by visiting the bank. However, great care must be taken to select the appropriate type of account (as explained next) for your situation and to assure that you have selected a trustworthy person to help you.

The following types of multiple-name accounts are commonly available:

Joint Account
In a joint account, any person whose name is on the account is considered a co-owner. Each named person can make deposits and withdrawals without the other person's knowledge or consent. There are a few facts about joint accounts to keep in mind:

- The other person could withdraw all of your money without consequence or legal recourse.
- The other person's creditors could tie up the funds in the account (with a lien or attachment) until proof of your ownership of the funds is provided.
- A person's name cannot be taken off the account without that person's written approval.
- In a joint account, when one owner dies, the survivor automatically owns the account without going through probate court. This can be a benefit because the funds are immediately available to pay urgent expenses, such as funeral costs. It can also have negative consequences if the joint account holder is not your intended beneficiary.

Authorized Signer Account
An authorized signer account, or a convenience account, allows another individual to make deposits and withdrawals to your

account and sign your checks. The other signer's creditors cannot tie up your account. However, as with joint accounts, there is still the risk that the other authorized signer could withdraw all your money from your account. Unlike a joint account, the account does not belong to the other authorized signer upon your death; rather, funds in this account belong to your estate—or to a named beneficiary (see later). The authority of the other signer ends with your death, so the other authorized signer will not be able to use the funds after your death.

Payable on Death Accounts and Beneficiary Designations

All checking, savings, investment, and retirement accounts allow you to designate to whom your account will be distributed at your death. Sometimes these accounts are called payable on death (POD) accounts. Both the beneficiary designation and the POD account allow for planning after your death, but these designations do not affect ownership during your life. The named beneficiary cannot make withdrawals or sign checks, so it is a useful way to bypass probate to give money to loved ones after your death.

Naming a Representative Payee

A representative payee is an individual or organization appointed by the U.S. Social Security Administration, the U.S. Office of Personnel Management, the U.S. Department of Veterans Affairs, or the U.S. Railroad Retirement Board who may be charged with receiving your income, using that income to pay your current expenses, saving for your future needs, and maintaining proper records. The Social Security Administration has a Representative Payee Program with rules and regulations to protect the beneficiary of the income. Learn more about the Representative Payee Program at http:// www.socialsecurity.gov/payee. To have the authority to manage your Social Security or Supplemental Security Income benefit, a person or organization must be appointed by the Social Security Administration. A power of attorney or note from you is not good enough. Having a representative appointed provides oversight that may give you assurance that your bills and finances will be properly handled. Many professional fiduciaries and organizations serve as representative payees.

Family Caregiving Contracts

Individuals are often uncomfortable with the idea of paying family members or friends for caregiving arrangements. But changes in the Medicaid asset transfer rules over the past 15 years, as well as the reality that caregivers must sometimes give up their day jobs in order to provide the necessary level of care, have made personal care contracts an attractive option, both to make sure that the level of care is met and that children (or other relatives or friends) do not have to sacrifice their own financial well-being while providing care to their parents.

Personal care contracts must, as a general rule, be in writing and state the kind and extent of services that are necessary, within reasonable terms. Because personal services contracts involve payment for services, income paid to a family caregiver through such a contract is subject to payroll and income taxes, and caregivers should consult an accountant to ensure that the income is reported properly. Tax credits are not available for parent caregiving unless the parent is the child's legal dependent.

Durable Power of Attorney

A power of attorney is an extremely important planning tool. It allows you to appoint someone to manage all of your financial affairs if you are unable to manage them yourself. If no power of attorney exists and it is necessary to liquidate or transfer assets or enter into real estate transactions (including those of a spouse), it may be necessary to go to court to establish a conservatorship before these matters can be acted on. Establishing a conservatorship can be costly and time-consuming. Thus, everyone should have a power of attorney.

Power of Attorney Defined

A **power of attorney** is a written document in which you (as the "principal") appoint another person (the "attorney-in-fact") to handle your property or finances. The power of attorney can be effective for all purposes or for a limited purpose (for example, appointing another person to sign a deed for the sale of your home when you are unavailable). A power of attorney becomes ineffective if the principal becomes incapacitated or dies.

Durable Power of Attorney Defined

A "durable" power of attorney continues to be valid even after the principal becomes incapacitated. A durable power of attorney document must specifically state that it is "durable" and must contain specific language, such as "This power of attorney shall continue to be effective if I become incapacitated or incompetent." Generally, if the purpose of a power of attorney is to make sure that someone can manage your finances when you cannot, the power of attorney should be durable.

Care Must Be Taken in Choosing an Attorney-in-Fact

Powers of attorney are not supervised by courts, so they can be abused if the wrong person is appointed attorney-in-fact. While the attorney-in-fact is required by law to act in the best interest of the principal, it is difficult to get your money back if the person you have appointed handles your affairs unwisely. Therefore, you must choose someone you trust implicitly—a person who will *always* act in your best interests.

Creating a Power of Attorney

While forms are available free on the Internet, it is best to consult an experienced attorney to create a power of attorney. Too many times, individuals sign documents they have printed off the Internet only to discover later that the documents are invalid or do not serve their purposes. This can be a very costly error, because it may be necessary to have a court appoint a conservator to do what could have been accomplished easily with a validly executed power of attorney.

Safeguards to Protect You

You may trust a friend or family member to be your attorney-in-fact and feel confident that no safeguards are necessary. However, another option is to hire a professional fiduciary, such as a bank trust department, to ensure that your finances are handled the way you want. Either way, consider including the following safeguards in a power of attorney:

- Require that the attorney-in-fact provide an annual or monthly accounting to you, your lawyer, an independent accountant, or a trusted family member to review.
- Name two attorneys-in-fact on the document and specify that they must act jointly (for example, both attorneys-in-fact must agree and both must sign checks).
- Require your appointed attorney-in-fact to obtain a surety bond to cover the value of your property if the attorney-in-fact mishandles your funds.
- Appoint a successor in case the attorney-in-fact dies, becomes incompetent, or simply chooses not to act on your behalf.

Cancelling or Ending a Power of Attorney

A power of attorney can be canceled or revoked at any time. Each state has specific requirements for revoking a power of attorney.

Your revocation should be sent to the attorney-in-fact and to any person or institution with whom the attorney-in-fact has done business on your behalf.

Remember, a power of attorney becomes invalid if the principal become incompetent or dies. However, a *durable* power of attorney continues if the principal becomes incompetent and can be revoked only by a guardian or conservator, if one has been appointed. A durable power of attorney terminates when the principal dies.

Trusts

A trust is a legal arrangement in which a person or a financial institution owns and manages assets for your benefit. The parties to a trust are the person setting up the trust (the "grantor"), the person or organization administering the trust (the "trustee"), and the person for whom the trust is established (the "beneficiary"). Often the grantor and the beneficiary are the same person.

An agreement, called a trust instrument, between the grantor and the trustee explains the trustee's authority. A trust can be created by the terms of the grantor's will (a **testamentary trust**) or during the grantor's lifetime (a **living trust**, also called an inter vivos trust). A living trust is the type of trust used to manage assets during a time of incapacity. Some trusts are court supervised, and some are not.

Trusts are not for everyone. A living trust is generally not appropriate for modest estates because the costs and disadvantages, including the time and logistics involved in administering them, outweigh the benefits. As with any planning tool, it is important to review each option for managing estates to determine the strategies that best fit your situation. In other words, one size does not fit all.

Basic Living Trust Defined

You may create a living trust during your lifetime by transferring ownership and control of your assets to the trust.

A trust can be revocable or irrevocable:

- As long as you are competent, you may change, revoke, or terminate a **revocable trust** at any time during your lifetime. A revocable trust is normally used for property management purposes. After you die, the revocable trust becomes irrevocable.
- A revocable living trust is often used as a planning tool because it allows a trustee to manage your property for your benefit during life and can also provide for distribution or ongoing management after your incapacity or death. Most commonly, in a living trust you would be both your own trustee and beneficiary. As such, your Social Security number would be used when establishing trust accounts or doing trust business. You would manage your property as if the property were in your name. A trust agreement would also include your directions should you become incompetent or die. If you have a medical condition that could result in your being unable to manage your affairs, a revocable living trust may be the right choice.
- An **irrevocable trust** cannot be changed or terminated after it has been established. It is a separate taxable entity, requiring its own tax identification number. Tax considerations may be a factor in deciding whether to make a trust revocable or irrevocable, particularly when a substantial amount of property is involved.

Care Must Be Taken in Choosing a Trustee

A trustee has as much, if not more, responsibility as an attorney-in-fact in a power of attorney. Great care must be taken in choosing your trustee. In most revocable living trusts, you would serve as trustee as long as you are able to do so. Should you become incapacitated, the "successor trustee" would take over and be responsible for management of all trust assets during your life and for distribution of those assets to the beneficiaries upon your death. Being a trustee is a huge responsibility and should not be taken lightly. While a family member or other individual could be named trustee if you are sure that person is trustworthy and capable of acting in this capacity, a fair amount of expertise is needed to handle the paperwork, tax returns, and property management tasks that may be involved. In most cities, professional trustees are available for hire, and many banking institutions have trust departments. Going over options with an attorney before naming a trustee is always wise.

Creating a Living Trust

A revocable living trust is established with the execution of a trust agreement. In this document, you would name the beneficiary (usually yourself during life), state how the property should be managed if you become disabled, and direct how the property should be distributed at your death. A living trust is much like a will in this way, and so many states require specific formalities in signing a

---

Important Tip

Be on guard against anyone who uses high-pressure tactics to sell a living trust package. Do not deal with anyone who demands a signature right away or requires money before you have time to do additional research. Some companies only want to sell their prepackaged plans and do not assist clients in putting assets into the trust. These trusts can cause problems that will be expensive to fix.

trust to ensure that you are not being coerced or unduly influenced by someone in executing the trust. Trusts should be drawn up by an attorney familiar with drafting them.

To receive the advantages of the revocable trust, all assets must be placed in the trust or the trust must be named beneficiary.

A Revocable Trust Cannot Be Used to Avoid Paying Nursing Home Costs

A revocable trust is considered an available resource under Medicaid laws and is not a way to avoid spending savings on nursing home care. The federal and state Medicaid laws are very complicated and subject to change at any time. Do not try to use a trust without getting competent legal advice.

Trusts for Protecting Assets While Dependent on Medicaid

People living with chronic conditions may ultimately require assistance with activities of daily living (ADLs), such as bathing, transferring, ambulation, eating, toileting, and basic hygiene and grooming. This type of assistance is known as custodial care. Individuals may receive this care at home, or they may need to move to an assisted living facility or a nursing home. No matter where these services are received, they are very expensive. Medicare does not cover the cost of custodial care. Long-term care insurance policies may cover these types of costs. However, it is difficult to obtain long-term care insurance after you are diagnosed with a significant medical condition. When long-term care insurance is not available, private funds must be used to pay for the cost of care. Once private funds are depleted, many individuals turn to Medicaid to pay for these services.

Medicaid eligibility rules are complex and vary depending on (among other things) the state in which you reside, whether you are married or single, the types of services you need, and your age. As a very general rule, however, you may keep a car and your home (as long as you are living in it) and about $3,000. Be aware that this amount varies from state to state. The point is, you can have only limited assets outside of your home and car. There are three types of trusts available that, if properly established and administered, allow a person with a disability to retain more than $3,000 and still be eligible for Medicaid to pay for the cost of care. These three trusts are a first-party special needs trust, a third-party special needs trust, and a pooled trust. The funds in any of these three trusts may be used to purchase goods and/or services that "supplement and do not supplant" government benefits. In other words, funds in the trust may be used for goods and/or services that benefit the individual and do not replace the government benefits the individual receives. For instance, funds may be used to pay for a companion dog, nonconventional treatments, massage, companion services, a home, rent, travel, or clothing. Funds may not be used to pay for medical services covered by Medicaid. Because you can have only $3,000 to be eligible for Medicaid to pay the cost of custodial care, having a special needs trust can make a significant difference in your life. Sometimes a special needs trust can make the difference between living at home or in a nursing home.

First-Party Special Needs Trust

A first-party special needs trust is a way for an individual to place his or her own money into a trust and remain eligible for Medicaid. It is called a "first-party" special needs trust because the individual's assets are used to fund the trust. Assets in a first-party special needs trust remain exempt if:

- The trust is established by a parent, grandparent, guardian, or court and is:
    - For the sole benefit of the person with the disability as certified by the Social Security Administration
    - For a person who is under the age of 65
    - Using the person's assets—this includes any assets a person may be awarded as a result of a personal injury lawsuit
- The trust is irrevocable by the beneficiary and may only be changed by the trustee if the change is necessary to comply with a new law or decision governing first-party special needs trusts.
- The trust has a provision that at the death of the person with the disability, any remaining trust assets must be distributed first to the state as repayment for any Medicaid that has been received.

Third-Party Special Needs Trust

A third-party special needs trust is a way for a third party to give money to a person with a disability in a way that does not jeopardize the individual's eligibility for public benefits. For instance, if a parent or grandparent or best friend wants to leave money to a person with a disability, or if friends want to throw a fundraiser, a third-party special needs trust is used. Sometimes third-party trusts are set up while the grantor is alive; other times they are set up in wills. Assets or funds belonging to the person with the disability must never be placed in the trust. There is no payback to the Medicaid Agency. Rather, the grantor may state who will receive any funds remaining in trust at the beneficiary's death. Laws regarding the supplemental needs trusts vary from state to state, and a lawyer should be consulted in each state.

Pooled Trust

A pooled trust is a type of special needs trust, and for all intents and purposes it is administered like a first-party special needs trust. However, a pooled trust must be established and managed by a nonprofit corporation. A separate subaccount must be maintained for each beneficiary of the trust, but, for purposes of investment and management, the trust pools the accounts. Each subaccount must be established solely for the benefit of individuals who are disabled as defined by the Social Security Administration. The subaccount may be set up by the parent, grandparent, or legal guardian of the individual, the individual him or herself, or by a court. To the extent that amounts remaining in the subaccount at the beneficiary's death are not retained by the pooled trust, the trust must pay such remaining amounts to the state in an amount equal to the total amount of Medicaid paid on behalf of the individual.

Health Care Directives

A **health care directive**, often called an advance directive, is a written document in which you appoint someone (a health care agent) to make health care decisions in the event you are unable to make them yourself.

A health care directive is now recognized as a combination of two earlier documents: the living will (a document that provides specific guidance to physicians, nurses, and caregivers about medical treatment) and a durable power of attorney for health care (a document that authorizes another person to make health care decisions when you are unable to do so).

Why Create a Health Care Directive?

You have the right to make decisions about your health care, including the right to refuse treatment, authorize treatment, and access information in your medical records. In a health care directive, you can authorize a trusted loved one, relative, or caregiver (the designated health care agent) to make necessary health care decisions according to your wishes if you are unable to do so yourself.

What Must a Health Care Directive Include?

Health care directives are governed by state law, and most state laws have several statutory requirements. Most important, a health care directive must be written by a competent person, and be dated, signed, and witnessed or notarized.

Who Can Be a Health Care Agent?

Your health care agent may be any individual 18 years of age or older who is not your health care provider or an employee of your health care provider. You should choose someone who you know well and trust to make decisions according to your wishes. It is very important to discuss your wishes in detail with a prospective health care agent before you finalize your decision. Make sure the person clearly understands your wishes *and* appreciates the responsibilities involved. You should also name a successor (backup) health care agent in case the primary health care agent is unable to act when decisions must be made.

What Is Included in the Health Care Directive?

In your health care directive, you may:

- Appoint one or more agents or alternative agents and include instructions for how decisions should be made and whether named agents must act together or may act independently

- State a preferred nursing home in the event such care is necessary
- State which medical records the health care agent can access
- State that the health care agent is the "personal representative" under the federal Health Insurance Portability and Accountability Act (HIPAA) and has the authority to access your medical records
- State whether the health care agent shall be guardian or conservator if a petition is filed
- State whether your eyes, tissues, or organs should be donated on your death
- Make a declaration regarding intrusive mental health treatment or a statement that the health care agent is authorized to give consent for such treatment
- State specific instructions if you are female and pregnant
- Give instructions regarding artificially administered nutrition or hydration
- State under what circumstances the health care directive will become effective
- State any other instructions regarding care, including how religious beliefs may affect health care delivery
- Provide instructions about being placed on a ventilator, receiving resuscitation, or other aggressive measures if there is minimal to no chance that you will recover
- State what will happen with your body at death (body identification/burial/cremation)

When Do the Health Care Agent's Responsibilities Begin?

Generally, the health care agent may make decisions for you when your physician believes you are unable to make your own decisions.

What Are the Duties of the Health Care Agent?

The health care agent is obligated to make informed, good-faith health care decisions from your point of view. The health care agent should follow your guidance in the health care directive and should seek legal help if the medical providers will not comply with his or her requests.

Can the Health Care Directive Be Cancelled or Revoked?

You may cancel or revoke the health care directive in whole or in part by:

- Destroying the document
- Executing a written and dated statement explaining what part of the health care directive you want to revoke
- Verbally expressing the intent to revoke it in the presence of witnesses
- Executing a new health care directive

Where Should the Health Care Directive Be Kept?

The health care directive must be readily available in an emergency. It should be kept with your personal papers in a safe place—such as your emergency notebook—(not in a safe deposit box unless someone else is also a signer on the box). You should give signed copies to family members, close friends, your health care agent, your backup health care agent, and your doctors so that they can include it in your medical records.

What Is the Uniform Anatomical Gift Act?

The Uniform Anatomical Gift Act allows you to donate your entire body, organs, tissues, or eyes for research or transplantation. If you do not make the gift, close relatives, a guardian, a conservator, or a health care agent may make an anatomical gift at the time of death—unless it is documented that you refused to donate organs while alive. Verification of intent to make an anatomical gift may be indicated on your driver's license.

Is a DNR/DNI/DNH the Same as a Health Care Directive?

The acronym DNR/DNI/DNH means "Do not resuscitate/do not intubate/do not hospitalize." This is a request by a patient to his or her physician to limit the scope of emergency medical care. The request is signed by the patient or the patient's proxy, and it must be ordered by a physician. It will be followed by emergency medical personnel if presented to them at the time of the emergency. You should have a health care directive as well, because the DNR/DNI/DNH is limited only to decisions regarding end of life and resuscitation or intubation and does not deal with all other myriad issues that may arise at the end of one's life.

What Is POLST and Is It the Same as a Health Care Directive?

POLST stands for Physician Orders for Life-Sustaining Treatment. It is an initiative that began in Oregon in 1991 in recognition that patient wishes for life-sustaining treatments were not being honored despite the availability of advance directives. POLST has endorsed programs in about 14 states and programs under development in many other states. It is a signed medical order that can be used by emergency medical technicians and other health care professionals during an emergency. The form is more specific than an advance directive and is signed by the patient's provider, making it a medical order. The physician must meet with the patient to go over the form and learn treatment options available for the specific disease or serious illness the patient has. Like the DNR/DNI/DNH order, POLST is not meant to take the place of an advance directive or the appointment of the agent.

Where Can I Obtain Health Care Directive Forms?

An attorney who specializes in eldercare law or has experience with health care directives can prepare a directive that is tailored to your needs.

In addition, suitable forms may be downloaded from reputable Web sites, such as the following:

- Aging with Dignity: http://www.agingwithdignity.org/five-wishes.php
- American Bar Association: http://www.abanet.org/publiced/practical/directive_whatis.html
- National Hospice and Palliative Care Organization: http://caringinfo.org/i4a/pages/index.cfm?pageid = 3289
- U.S. Living Wills Registry: http://liv-will1.uslivingwillregistry.com/forms.html
- The Departments of Health in individual states

Guardianship and Conservatorship

Guardianships and conservatorships are relationships between two people created by the court to protect people who cannot handle their own financial or personal affairs. Definitions vary from state to state. Most generally, a **guardian** is appointed for the purpose of managing the personal affairs of a person who has become incapacitated (called a ward), including making personal decisions and meeting needs for medical care, nutrition, clothing, shelter, or safety. A **conservator** is appointed for a person (called a protected person) for the purpose of managing finances, assets, and income when it has been shown that the person has impaired ability and/ or judgment. If a person needs both a guardian and a conservator, one person may be appointed by the court to fill both of those roles.

A Guardianship or Conservatorship Is Required When No Plan Is in Place

A guardianship or conservatorship is necessary when a person becomes unable to handle finances or live safely without help and no previous arrangements have been made. The decision to obtain a guardianship or conservatorship should not be made lightly because it takes away the person's most basic right: to make decisions about his or her own health and welfare. The court will appoint a guardian or conservator who will handle all of the person's affairs, including perhaps where he or she will live.

The court will appoint a guardian or conservator only if a less restrictive alternative is not available for managing the personal and financial affairs of the person. It is likely that no guardianship or conservatorship will be necessary if a health care directive and a power of attorney have been put into place.

It is likely that neither a guardianship nor conservatorship will be necessary if a health care directive and a power of attorney have been put into place.

Establishment of a Guardianship or Conservatorship

While practices may vary state by state, generally a guardianship or conservatorship is established by filing a petition with the probate court in the county where the person resides. Anyone can ask the court to appoint a guardian or conservator for a person who needs help. The potential ward or protected person must be given advance notice of the hearing and has the right to be represented by an attorney at any court proceeding, even if he or she cannot pay for the attorney. In this case, the court will order the county to pay these costs. The person requesting a guardianship or conservatorship must prove through clear and convincing evidence that such an order is necessary. This could be difficult if the proposed ward or protected person does not want a guardianship or conservatorship established.

Your Will

A **will** is a set of written instructions about how to dispose of your assets upon death. Assets are either described as probate assets or nonprobate assets. Probate assets are those assets whose ownership a court must rule on following the owner's death. Nonprobate assets are assets that will automatically transfer to another person at death such as those with joint tenancy or beneficiary designations or assets that have been placed in a trust. Probate court is the court charged with determining ownership either by administering a legal will or by state law when no legal will exists.

Not Everyone Needs a Will—But It Is a Good Idea

If property is held in such a way that it will pass through beneficiary designations or joint ownership, then a will is not technically necessary. However, a will is necessary if a person wants personal property, such as jewelry, paintings, and family heirlooms, distributed in a certain way. Tax or private family matters may exist that make it wise to use a will and probate court to administer an estate. Finally, even if there seems to be no reason for a will, having one is the best way to ensure that an individual's wishes will be followed.

PART 3

What Can I and My Medical
Team Do About It?

Chapter 8

Benign Tumors

This chapter focuses on tumors within the skull but outside of the brain. Such tumors are usually found by accident, such as during screening for a head injury, and tend to be benign, or not cancerous. However, depending on the tumor's location, its effects may not be benign at all. Benign brain tumors may cause significant neurologic damage. For most meningiomas, pituitary adenomas, and acoustic neuromas, watchful waiting is the name of the game. In many cases, the tumor can be removed by a neurosurgeon and will never recur. In others, the tumor can have a menacing course, requiring multiple surgeries, radiation treatment, and, in rare instances, chemotherapy.

"If you have to have a brain tumor, this is the one to have."
That's what Lynn was told by doctors when she found herself faced with meningioma. A bout of arm and leg pain she suspected was shingles brought her to the local emergency room, where she received the diagnosis. And though she isn't exactly recommending the experience, Lynn has nothing but good things to say.

Turns out, Lynn's pains were unrelated to the tumor, which was benign. Nonetheless, she elected to have the tumor removed as it rested against a vein, a danger if it were to grow. Lynn barraged her medical team with questions: How do you get the skull back on? Can I still go through airport security? The answers were a comfort. "I really, honestly, was not that nervous," she says, adding with a laugh,

"I watch Grey's Anatomy." Now, *she endures the screws in her* head, *but has devised a hairstyle to conceal them.*

In this chapter, you will learn the following:

- **What meningioma, pituitary adenoma, and acoustic neuroma are**
- **About their symptoms and treatment options**
- **What stereotactic radiosurgery is and how it's used**
- **What radiation necrosis is and how it's treated**
- **How having one of these tumors types might affect your life**

Basics About Meningioma

A meningioma is a tumor that arises from the covering of the brain, or the meninges. Meningiomas are the most common tumors that occur within the skull. They are considered benign, or slow growing. In most cases, a meningioma is found incidentally. An individual may have hit his or her head or may have been injured in a car accident, prompting a computerized tomography (CT) scan that reveals the abnormality. Meningiomas sometimes occur in the context of rare genetic syndromes, such as neurofibromatosis, and also result from prior radiation exposure to the head and spine.

On a CT scan with contrast dye, a meningioma typically shows a sharply defined border compared to normal brain tissue (Figure 8–1). It is frequently identified by the presence of a small tail of tissue called a "dural tail" where it attaches to the dura, or coverings, of the brain. Meningiomas come in many sizes, some so large they produce brain swelling and very significant neurologic problems, and others so tiny that they may be difficult to detect. In some cases, meningiomas develop areas of calcification, or hardening, because of collections of psammoma bodies, or rounded

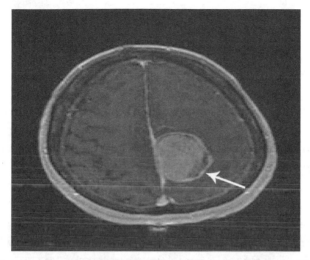

Figure 8-1 Axial view of the brain (feet up) showing a meningioma.

collections of calcium within the tumor. They may also be enveloped by bony growth or cause the overlying skull to erode. When viewed after the injection of contrast dye, a meningioma picks up the contrast uniformly and is clearly defined from the surrounding brain tissue.

Because meningiomas are so slow growing, the brain typically makes room for them; as a result, many patients report experiencing few or no symptoms. Nevertheless, in some patients the tumors exert pressure on certain areas of the brain, causing headache, blurred vision, numbness, seizures, eye-movement difficulties, or trouble with hearing, speech, or swallowing. When they occur along the spine, meningiomas can cause back pain, weakness, balance difficulty, and bowel and bladder trouble.

In cases without neurologic symptoms, a conservative treatment approach includes monitoring the meningioma with regular magnetic resonance imaging (MRI) or CT scans. If the tumor has begun to cause symptoms, a neurosurgeon will determine whether the safe removal of the entire tumor or a portion of it is possible.

Interestingly, certain tumors often resemble meningiomas in their imaging appearance. Common mimickers include metastases (tumors spread to the brain from elsewhere in the body); hemangiopericytoma, a rare tumor that arises from the same cells as a meningioma; or solitary fibrous tumors. When a meningioma mimic is suspected, either because of an atypical imaging appearance or rapid growth, surgery is often advised.

Although most meningiomas are benign, some have proved frustratingly persistent. Take the case of Rhett, a fourth-generation pharmacist, for example. "My head is loaded with them," he says. After a massive seizure sent Rhett to the emergency room in 1992, a CT scan of his skull revealed atypical meningiomas "the size of walnuts." "My family doctor said, 'I have good news and bad. You've got brain tumors— four, maybe five. The good news? They're operable, a superficial type that haven't penetrated into the brain tissue." Since then, Rhett has weathered numerous surgeries, radiation treatment, and chemotherapy and continues to have yearly neurologic checkups.

The diagnosis "walloped me," he says. But his faith in the support, love, and pie-baking skills of his wife, Jane; in his doctors; and in staying positive has kept Rhett in good spirits. "I'm a very religious man," he says. "My prayer has been answered."

Treating Atypical and Malignant Meningiomas

Although most meningiomas are benign, some are fast growing and tend to recur; such tumors are called atypical. In cases where the cells are rapidly dividing and developing their own blood supply, the meningioma is considered to be malignant. On MRI, the only clue that a meningioma is atypical or malignant is the presence of surrounding brain irritation or direct brain invasion. Despite these common imaging features, the neurosurgeon will need to obtain tissue for the pathologist to review.

In some cases, if the location of the mass makes surgery difficult, another option is stereotactic radiosurgery (SRS). Contrary to its name, SRS is not surgery at all. Instead, SRS describes the one-time use of a focused beam of high-dose radiation directed at the tumor. SRS is most successful on well-defined lesions or tumors that measure less than 3 centimeters around (the size of a walnut or smaller). During this procedure, the neurosurgeon places a frame on the patient's head to ensure proper alignment for the SRS treatment, which is administered by a radiation oncologist.

Most patients do well with SRS. One significant side effect, however, is **radiation necrosis**, which describes the death of brain tissue. The treatment for radiation necrosis typically involves the use of steroids. For cases that steroid use fails to improve, the necrotic tissue may have to be removed by surgery. Currently, researchers are evaluating the effectiveness of several other treatments against radiation necrosis, including hyperbaric oxygen, pentoxifylline, vitamin E, and bevacizumab.

After surgical removal of a meningioma, the patient will undergo periodic follow-up testing on MRI or CT scans to monitor the tumor site. If the tumor recurs, a second surgery is an option. If more surgery is considered too risky, however, or if a large amount of tumor is left behind (larger than 3 centimeters), a radiation oncologist will treat the remaining tumor using 4–6 weeks of conventional radiation therapy.

Research into the effectiveness of treating meningiomas with chemotherapy remains inconclusive. Various agents, including hydroxyurea and a combination of cyclophosphamide, doxorubicin (Adriamycin), and vincristine (CAV), have been tested without significant results. If you're interested in exploring clinical trials, ask your treating neurologist/medical oncologist to inform you about any opportunities and your possible eligibility to participate in these trials.

Pituitary Adenoma

The pituitary gland is attached to the brain and lies within the base of the skull. It secretes various hormones that control human growth, lactation, thyroid function, and adrenaline. Occasionally, pituitary tissue can grow in an uncontrolled fashion. The resulting tumor is called a **pituitary adenoma**. Such tumors are visible on a CT scan or MRI performed either with or without the injection of contrast dyes (Figure 8–2). Depending on the size of the patient's pituitary gland, it is classified either as a microadenoma, about the size of a pea (10 millimeters or smaller), or a macroadenoma, roughly the size of a lima bean (larger than 10 millimeters).

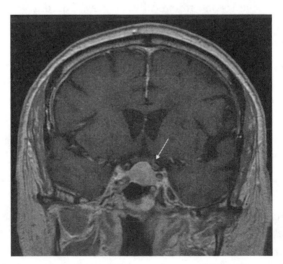

Figure 8–2 Arrow is pointing to a typical appearing pituitary adenoma.

Typically, when a pituitary adenoma is found incidentally, the individual is referred to a neurologist, a neuro-oncologist, or an endocrinologist (a doctor who specializes in hormones). After the doctor takes a careful history and physical exam, the patient is sent to an ophthalmologist, a doctor who specializes in the eyes, for visual-field testing. Such testing helps determine whether any loss of peripheral vision has occurred. The doctor may also order specialized MRIs to take a closer look at the pituitary mass, in addition to blood work to determine whether the tumor is secreting any hormones. Once clear images of the mass are in hand, the doctor and patient will discuss any symptoms the tumor may be causing.

Functioning and Nonfunctioning Pituitary Adenomas

Pituitary adenomas are classified in two ways: functioning, meaning the cells are secreting hormones, or nonfunctioning, meaning no hormone secretion is taking place. Many patients with a nonfunctioning pituitary adenoma have no symptoms, and the tumor is discovered accidentally, though this is generally true for tumors with dimensions of less than 10 millimeters. Indeed, as the tumor size increases, the likelihood that the patient has symptoms also rises. Symptoms include headache and disturbance in peripheral vision. The pituitary gland is also near blood vessels that supply and drain the brain. Tumor invasion of this area (called the cavernous sinus) causes symptoms such as headaches, trouble with eye movements, and strokes.

Patients with a functioning pituitary adenoma often experience a wide range of symptoms. Such symptoms include thyroid dysfunction, which can cause intolerance to heat or cold, weight gain or loss, or hair growth or loss; lactation (the secretion or production of milk in the mammary glands); and **acromegaly,** a condition in which an excessive amount of growth hormone can result in an enlarged lower jaw, hands, or feet. Certain medications may be used to shrink the pituitary adenoma or to counteract those hormones. If the tumor's size is beginning to intrude upon or dam-age nearby structures, the doctor will refer the patient to a neuro-surgeon and possibly to a radiation oncologist. Depending on the type of hormone secreted, a pituitary tumor may take on a different name. For example, if a pituitary tumor secretes a hormone called prolactin, the tumor is called a prolactinoma. For prolactinomas, certain medications, including bromocriptine, pergolide, and cab-ergoline, work well to shrink the tumor. A panel of screening blood tests will help determine how well the tumor will respond to such medications.

Treatment Paths

If the tumor is small, nonfunctioning, and not secreting any hormones: The tumor will typically be monitored with serial MRI scans and visual-field testing. Any change, even a subtle one, is likely to be detected first by a change in the size or shape of the mass as seen on MRI, or a change in the visual field, often before any abnormal-ity is noticed by the patient.

If the tumor is large, secreting hormones, and/or is causing significant symptoms: A neurosurgeon will determine whether the tumor can and should be safely removed. Such procedures occasionally require the ex-pertise of an otolaryngologist (an ear, nose, and throat doctor) as the pituitary gland can be accessed through the sinus. Otherwise, a neuro-surgeon may perform a biopsy to confirm the pathology.

Surgery

Patients who are candidates for surgery will be prescribed corticos-teroids in the periods before and after the operation to reduce the risk of hormonal dysregulation, or disruption, should the pituitary gland become damaged during surgery. Sodium levels in the blood and urine will also be monitored to maintain the body's normal salt-water balance. Postsurgery, if the pituitary gland remains intact, a patient may not require supplemental hormones. If, on the other hand, the pituitary gland is removed in its entirety, the individual will require supplemental hormones, such as cortisone, testosterone, and/or estrogen, under the supervision of an endocrinologist.

If a surgical procedure is deemed too risky, radiation therapy remains an option. A radiation oncologist will oversee the individual's care in an effort to halt the growth of the tumor and to promote its shrinkage.

Acoustic Neuroma

Acoustic neuromas, also called vestibular schwannomas, are benign tumors found in the small angle in the brain between the cerebellum and the pons, part of the brainstem, and arise from the eighth cranial nerve (the hearing and balance nerve) as it exits the brainstem. The eighth cranial nerve provides input for hearing and balance and helps coordinate eye movements. An acoustic neuroma sometimes is discovered incidentally on a CT scan or MRI, or may be suspected when a patient reports hearing loss in one ear, trouble with walking and balance, or vertigo. Depending on the location, additional symptoms may occur, such as Bell's palsy, facial pain, and weakness on the opposite side of the body. Acoustic neuromas are more common in women than in men.

Acoustic neuromas tend to occur on one side of the brain or the other. Those observed on both sides of the brain may indicate an underlying genetic syndrome called neurofibromatosis type 2, which runs in families and causes unusual skin tumors and other types of brain tumors in addition to acoustic neuromas. Upon detecting a tumor that looks like an acoustic neuroma, the neurologist and neurosurgeon will carefully examine the patient as well as refer her or him for hearing testing. If the patient is asymptomatic, meaning without symptoms, the tumor will be followed on a regular interval with MRI scans. However, if the patient reports symptoms, surgery and/or radiation treatment is among the recommended protocol. Typically, surgery is reserved for patients who have either lost their hearing or suffered significant neurologic damage related to the tumor's growth. The surgeon must then determine whether the tumor can be removed. In cases where the tumor is intertwined with the hearing nerve, the main risk of surgery is complete hearing loss. And because the hearing nerve and the nerve that controls facial expressions are closely related, damage to the facial nerve is another possible surgical risk.

If the risks of surgery are too great, radiation therapy remains another possibility. Radiation does not typically reverse neurologic damage; instead, it is used to stop its progression. The radiation oncologist may opt to treat the tumor with SRS, a one-time dose of intense, focused-beam radiation. This treatment may be appropriate if the tumor appears to be well defined and measures less than 3 centimeters. The risks of radiation include further damage to the hearing nerve, leading to hearing loss, and damage to nearby structures such as the facial nerve and brainstem.

How Will Having One of These Tumors Affect My Life?

As you can see, there are many different variables involved in the diagnosis and treatment of benign brain tumors. Some individuals, like Lynn, will experience relatively few if any symptoms and may even be able to avoid more invasive treatments. The lucky ones, after a successful course of treatment, will remain tumor-free for the remainder of their lives.

Others, like Rhett, will embark on a journey of repeated surgeries and radiation therapy. Their lives will be punctuated with frequent visits to their medical team for monitoring. Complex cases can prompt an abrupt change of lifestyle and a reranking of personal priorities. In Rhett's case, he was forced to retire from a long career in the pharmacy profession. At the same time, retirement allowed him to divide the year between homes in Arizona and Wisconsin, never far from the watchful eye of his medical team.

Because these tumors are benign, once a patient adjusts to the symptoms, life can go on as before. People with a pituitary adenoma should face few limitations as long as they take hormone supplements to replace the inactive or missing pituitary, while their endocrinologist monitors and "fine-tunes" these medications. People with acoustic neuroma will have more significant problems, particularly with hearing and control of facial muscles. Many will live with permanent weakness on the side of the face where the tumor was removed. This can cause concerns about personal appearance as well as trouble with eating and slurring of speech. As a result, people with acoustic neuroma should think carefully about their choice for radiation therapy or surgery. It's a good idea to get several opinions before committing to a plan of care.

Chapter 9

Primary Brain Tumors

Sometimes, an individual's access to medical information is no match for helpful, thoughtful context and guidance. A bout of bad headaches and facial and arm numbness led Shiy to seek medical help. She soon felt in over her head.

"When I first heard the pathology results, to be honest, I was like, 'What?'" she recalls. "My surgeon told me, 'Don't listen to the statistics. Everyone's different. Keep your chin up.'"

She was confused about what he was telling her. "I had no idea it meant cancer," she says. "After a couple of days, I started thinking, Statistics? Why's he telling me this?" Shiy went online and typed in the diagnosis she had received of anaplastic astrocytoma. When she read that people with that type of brain tumor had a survival rate of 2 to 3 years, "I completely freaked out," she says.

To enter the world of treatment of brain tumors is to travel to a completely foreign land. Many words you will hear are strange acronyms, like MRI (magnetic resonance imaging, a method to detect tumor growth), "Cat" scan (computerized tomography, abbreviated "CT scan," a type of skull X-ray), or GBM (glioblastoma multiforme, an advanced form of the tumor astrocytoma). You're out of your comfort zone. Emotions are raw. Events often move forward at a rapid pace, with scans and even surgery scheduled within days.

This chapter is intended to help slow things down for you—to give you an opportunity to read and digest things at your own pace.

According to experts in diagnosing and treating primary brain tumors (tumors that originate in the brain), a patient's long-term survival depends upon three main factors: (1) age, (2) how well the tumor responds to treatment, and (3) tumor type. Younger people tend to have an increased survival rate, as do those who are active and able to care for themselves. In general, those with grade 1 tumors have a better prognosis than those with grade 4 tumors. (The grading system is explained in depth later in this chapter.)

Also, the successful surgical removal of a tumor can make a difference in long-term survival. Most malignant primary brain tumors eventually grow back, often in the original location. The more tumor that can be surgically removed, the longer before the tumor reappears, and the better the prognosis. Surgery is generally followed by radiation therapy and chemotherapy. Yes, it *is* brain surgery, so there are many important factors to consider.

In this chapter, you will learn the following:

- **The treatment options you have**
- **How biopsy and surgery differ**
- **The advantages and disadvantages of each approach**
- **What role genetics plays in recovery**
- **How to read and understand pathology reports**
- **How radiation therapy and chemotherapy work**
- **What a clinical trial is**

Understanding Your Treatment Options

For primary brain tumors, a complete cure—meaning the tumor is gone, never to return—is rare. In most instances, the tumor will recur. Therefore, it is important to make treatment decisions relatively quickly and to employ the best available treatment options. Many people with brain tumors need treatment from a medical team that includes radiation oncologists, neuro-oncologists, rehabilitation specialists, and neurosurgeons. If possible, seek out a center that routinely cares for brain tumor patients. A team-oriented care philosophy can improve the outcome of treatment. Cases are often reviewed by a committee, or tumor board, composed of specialists from various disciplines to help determine the best treatment options.

A Few Thoughts About Choosing a Neurosurgeon

In general, some neurosurgeons specialize in spinal surgery and others in cranial, or brain, surgery. The most important thing is to work with an experienced tumor surgeon. Neurosurgeons operate on 30 to 200 brain tumor patients per year, and no "magic number" establishes competence. Neurosurgeons at larger facilities, such as multidisciplinary clinics or university medical centers, will often have more experience, and they may also have younger residents in their training programs helping them in the operating room. As a result, patients may benefit from the extra attention they receive from a care team informed with the latest training. On the other hand, you may be more comfortable choosing an experienced surgeon who prefers to do surgeries without young trainees at her or his side.

You should feel comfortable asking all specialists involved in your care questions about their experience and results in treating other patients with similar problems. It is crucial that you and your caregivers be well informed regarding the treatment choices and associated risks and benefits.

Surgery

Your neurosurgeon takes many different factors into account during the evaluation stage. The general health and neurologic condition of the patient are important concerns. Other factors, such as tumor location, the likely diagnosis based on imaging, and the depth of the tumor, will influence the relative risk of surgery.

Technological advances in imaging, surgical technique, and the delivery of therapeutic radiation have expanded options for patients with brain tumors. Your neurosurgeon will discuss those options with you, as well as the relative advantages and disadvantages of each one, to develop the best treatment approach.

Many patients with a brain tumor will need a biopsy before surgery. The exceptions are patients who have a relatively small, benign-appearing tumor. These individuals may be candidates for stereotactic (focused) radiation and thus may avoid invasive surgery.

Needle biopsy describes a procedure in which a tiny sample of the tumor tissue is obtained via a small opening in the skull, or **burr hole**, created using a specialized drill. A needle is then directed along a very precise path assisted by a computer program that guides the needle in three dimensions. This method allows the surgeon to sample the tissue very precisely. A pathologist then evaluates the sample under a microscope to confirm the exact cell type and grade of the tumor. The diagnosis depends upon this information. Based on these findings, your doctors will review the treatment options, such as chemotherapy and/or radiation, with you.

A biopsy is a minimally invasive procedure; it's relatively quick, taking about an hour. The biopsy helps with diagnosis but does not help the patient improve, since only a very small sample of the tumor is obtained. There is a risk that the sample may not accurately reflect the tumor type since it is sampled "blindly." A biopsy is not advisable in all situations. There are some circumstances, such as when a tumor has infiltrated the brainstem, in which the surgical procedure might result in new neurologic problems, including paralysis or double vision.

Of course, any surgery of the brain should be undertaken with great care, and results vary depending on many different factors. Charlie, whose wife, Pamela, died of a grade 4 glioblastoma multiforme, recalls feeling ill prepared for the unintended side effects of his wife's biopsy. "She went in a fully functional woman," he says. "She came out paralyzed on the left side. She was incapable of doing things on her own."

A biopsy is more often considered in people who are medically frail and for those in situations where removing the tumor is likely to increase the risk of worsening the individual's neurologic condition. This is true when the tumor has infiltrated into a part of the brain that cannot successfully be removed without making the patient worse, such as the primary motor control of the arm or leg. If the tumor has infiltrated into the frontal lobe or the temporal lobe, these areas can usually be removed more completely without affecting the neurologic functioning of the patient.

The risks of a brain biopsy include stroke, infection, bleeding, and the possibility of obtaining an inadequate specimen for diagnosis. Fortunately, modern techniques have dramatically reduced the risk of these complications. Many patients leave the hospital on the day of the biopsy or the following morning. Thanks to modern imaging and surgical techniques, many individuals now leave the hospital within a few days of surgery. Pain from the incision, or surgical wound, is typically controlled with mild oral medication. Patients are often amazed at how well they feel after brain surgery. Since there are no pain fibers within the brain itself, and because there has been no abdominal or chest incision to impede digestion or breathing, craniotomy patients are mobile very quickly after the procedure. Incisions can usually be placed behind the hairline to minimize the visibility of scarring after the incision has healed. Rigid plates are used to secure the bone opening to the rest of the skull to prevent scalp deformity.

Resection describes the surgical removal of a tumor, which is accomplished through a procedure called a **craniotomy**. A craniotomy involves removing a piece of the skull to access the brain. After the tumor is either partially removed (**debulked**) or totally removed (**resected**), the bone is usually put back into place. The patient is under anesthesia during this procedure, which lasts several hours depending on the tumor's location. Family members can usually visit within a few hours of surgery. Resections can be further classified. A gross total resection means all apparent abnormal tissue has been removed and a repeat MRI will not show any residual tumor. A **subtotal resection** means some, but not all, of the tumor was removed, and a repeat MRI will show some residual tumor.

Advances in imaging, such as MRI, and improved surgical techniques have substantially improved the risks and recovery following removal of a brain tumor. Navigation, or frameless **stereotaxy**, allows the surgeon to use a scan taken before surgery and with the assistance of a global positioning system–like device to approach the tumor through a smaller bone opening and to guide its removal. Sometimes a patient's neurologic function will be monitored if the tumor is close to nerves leaving the brain or is in an "eloquent" region, or in especially delicate areas of the brain. Such areas can also be brain mapped with preoperative imaging or during surgery—in a process involving small electrodes attached to the brain—while the patient is kept awake through specialized anesthetic techniques. In brain mapping, the patient is required to talk, count, and perform other basic tasks during surgery to improve the surgeon's accuracy.

The decision to proceed with a resection isn't necessarily easy or straightforward. As discussed in Chapter 1, much of the decision depends on the tumor's location. Primary brain tumors are infiltrative, meaning tumor cells are intermingled among normal brain cells; thus, it is impossible to remove a tumor without damaging some normal brain tissue as well. In most cases, the risks of surgery must be weighed against the benefits. For instance, it may not be worth jeopardizing the patient's ability to walk, talk, and care for himself or herself. As a consequence, the decision to biopsy or resect a tumor is made with much thought and concern by the person with the brain tumor, his or her caregivers, and the neurosurgeon.

Technological advancements have expanded the range of tumors that can be operated upon within reasonable risk tolerances. Of course, such methods do not replace careful surgical judgment and skill. Brain surgery does have risks, such as bleeding, infection, and increased neurologic handicap. Your surgeon should discuss with you the specifics of your surgery, its risks, and the anticipated postoperative course, as well as nonsurgical options.

The main benefit of surgery is the significant relief of symptoms many patients experience within a few days of the operation. Complete surgical removal of the tumor may result in a cure for patients with benign brain tumors. Those with high-grade (fast-growing) primary brain tumors typically experience a better quality of life after surgery before they proceed with radiation and/or chemotherapy.

After surgery some individuals experience a temporary worsening of their neurologic function, which is caused by brain swelling. Typically, they are placed on steroids to minimize brain swelling. While in the hospital after surgery, patients are carefully monitored for signs of brain swelling and bleeding. Most postoperative neurologic impairments will improve substantially with time and rehabilitation.

Some patients, especially those with primary brain tumors that continue to grow after initial treatment, are candidates for repeat surgery. Another option is a second course of radiation. Further options, such as placing small catheters around the tumor to infuse medication, are currently under investigation, as are newer biological agents and individualized therapies based on certain DNA rearrangements within the tumors. Your treatment team will discuss the various options available to you if your tumor is progressing.

For 2 years, Peggy had written off her ever-worsening head-aches as hormonal, until she was diagnosed with a grade 3 oligodendroglioma of the left frontal lobe. She had an MRI on a Friday and surgery the following Wednesday. "I had a complete surgical excision," she says. "I was elated when I woke up. I could speak and move my extremities. I felt like myself."

Her postsurgical treatment took the classic form of a 6-week course of combined radiation therapy and chemotherapy. The regimen was "fatiguing," she adds, "but having a 2–1/2-year-old, I don't know which is more exhausting."

Understanding Your Pathology Report

Gliomas come in two basic types and four different grades (see Table 9–1). These criteria are accepted internationally. Once a tissue sample has been obtained, either through a biopsy (sampling of tissue) or a resection (surgical removal of a portion of or the entire tumor), a pathologist will examine your tumor under the microscope and provide an exact diagnosis.

Table 9–1 Tumor Types and Grades

Tumor Type	Grade I	Grade II	Grade III	Grade IV
Oligodendroglioma		Low-grade glioma (LGG)	Anaplastic oligodendroglioma (AO)	
Astrocytoma	Pilocytic astrocytoma	Low-grade glioma (LGG)	Anaplastic astrocytoma (AA)	Glioblastoma multiforme (GBM)
Oligoastrocytoma		Low-grade glioma (LGG)	Anaplastic oligoastrocytoma (AOA)	

Based on the characteristic appearance of the tissue, your tumor will be called an oligodendroglioma or an astrocytoma—or, on occasion, a combination of both, an oligoastrocytoma. Your report will also designate a grade, reflecting the tumor's aggressiveness. Grade 1 is the least aggressive and, in most cases, can be cured with resection. Grade 4 is the most aggressive and has a poorer prognosis. In some cases, a grade may alter the way in which a tumor is normally referred. For instance, a grade 4 astrocytoma is known as glioblastoma multiforme. Alternately, doctors may describe a grade 3 oligodendroglioma or astrocytoma as **anaplastic**, which means it is malignant. To determine a grade, the pathologist considers a few key features of the tumor sample: the presence or absence of cellularity, mitoses, vascular proliferation, and necrosis. **Cellularity** describes whether an excess of cells is present, such that the tissue does indeed resemble a tumor mass. **Mitoses**, or mitotic figures, refers to the various phases of cellular division, indicating that the tumor is growing and dividing. The test commonly used to determine the presence of mitoses is known as the **KI-67 stain**, a sensitive way to measure rapidly dividing cells, which might be listed on your report. (Less than 5 percent staining generally indicates a more benign tumor, while more than 5 percent staining is seen in more aggressive tumors.) Tumors are able to grow and support themselves through the development of new blood vessels, a process called **vascular proliferation**. Once vascular proliferation is identified, a grade will increase to a 3 or 4. Lastly, the pathologist looks for **necrosis**, or dead tissue, in certain parts of the tumor as well as in the underlying brain.

As you learn to read and understand your pathology report, after the grade and cell type (e.g., grade 3 oligodendroglioma) you may find other numbers and letters indicating **genetic markers**. These hereditary factors provide further information about your tumor type and the likelihood of it responding to certain treatments. For example, recent research shows that patients who lack two particular chromosomes—1p and 19q—in their tumor's genetic makeup are more likely to respond successfully to treatment. Another marker now being measured on an experimental basis is methylguanine-DNA methyltransferase (MGMT). If MGMT is inactivated, a patient's DNA cannot repair itself, which appears to improve the efficacy of chemotherapy regimens. One further marker, the P53 gene, located on chromosome 17, has been shown to suppress the development of tumors. Damage to this gene (as in people with Li-Fraumeni cancer syndrome) impairs the body's suppression response to the development of tumors; therefore, these patients have an increased number and type of cancers.

Radiation Therapy and Chemotherapy

Based on the grade and cell type of your tumor, treatment options range from careful observation with frequent MRI scans, to the use of oral chemotherapy, to a combination of both radiation therapy followed by oral chemotherapy. Discussed in detail in Chapter 3, radiation therapy is planned and administered by a radiation oncologist, and chemotherapy is prescribed by a neuro-oncologist or medical oncologist.

Radiation therapy, a treatment that uses high-energy X-rays or other types of ionizing radiation to prevent the division of cancer cells, does not hurt. The most common side effects are hair loss over the scalp portion corresponding to the tumor location, along with fatigue. The actual sessions are quite brief; you may find it takes longer to drive to the center and park in the lot than it does to receive the treatment. During the radiation portion of your treatment, you will be seen daily, Monday through Friday, by a member of the radiation team. Your neuro-oncologist or medical oncologist will visit with you at least at the initiation and completion of your radiation and also commonly midway through treatment to perform periodic blood tests.

Chemotherapy is a regimen of anticancer drugs taken by mouth. Currently, a drug called temozolomide (brand name: Temodar®) is the gold standard of treatment (the best possible treatment) for grade 4 astrocytomas, or glioblastoma multiforme. Temozolomide is an oral chemotherapy frequently prescribed in conjunction with radiation therapy for grade 3 and grade 4 gliomas. It works to disrupt the DNA of tumor cells. Following initial diagnosis, temozolomide is taken daily over approximately 6 weeks of radiation therapy. It is fairly well tolerated, with constipation, nausea, fatigue, and, in some cases, drop in blood counts (bone marrow suppression) as its most common side effects. In many cases, patients report feeling as though they are not taking chemotherapy at all.

Once the radiation portion of treatment is complete, a dosage of temozolomide is taken 5 days per month for the following 6 to 12 months, presuming the patient responds well and can tolerate it. During that second, or adjuvant, phase of treatment, an MRI is typically performed every other month to determine whether the tumor is continuing to respond to treatment. As long as the tumor is responding positively, the patient and medical team may agree to stop chemotherapy while continuing to follow up with regularly scheduled MRI scans. If the tumor looks like it is growing back or recurring, a decision is made to attempt more surgery, to turn to other chemotherapies, or to consider a clinical trial.

Clinical trials follow federal research guidelines to evaluate new drug treatments or devices. Data are collected during the clinical trial to evaluate the safety and efficacy of the new treatment. The latest result with positive outcomes becomes the next gold standard for therapy. Clinical trials are described in phases. Progression from one phase to the next depends upon the success of the previous phase.

- Phase I trials are small, most often involving fewer than 30 patients, and are typically conducted at only one institution.

They gauge whether a treatment is safe enough to proceed
with additional testing.

- Phase II trials assess whether a treatment found safe during the Phase I trial is effective against a particular type of
cancer.
- Phase III trials study whether a treatment is more effective
than the already established gold standard. Phase III trials involve hundreds of patients and are conducted by large
organizations nationwide.

Patients often ask their neuro-oncologists to recommend the
"best" clinical trial. However, when a trial is ongoing, we don't
yet have the answer. Once the trial is completed, if the treatment is shown to be better, it becomes the new standard of care.
Patients who enroll in clinical trials need to understand these
fundamental facts. They are enrolling to advance science and,
hopefully, to increase our understanding of brain tumor treatments. But they will likely not directly benefit from being a par-
ticipant in a trial.

Fortunately, new options continue to emerge for the treatment
of recurrent gliomas. One promising new approach that targets
angiogenesis, or the tumor's ability to make and sustain its own
blood vessels, is **bevacizumab** (an antivascular endothelial growth
factor or anti-VEGF agent whose brand name is Avastin). It is an
intravenous monoclonal antibody administered twice monthly
that has been approved by the US Food and Drug Administration
(FDA) for use in recurrent glioblastoma. Apart from some rare side
effects, such as high blood pressure, clotting, and colon damage, it
is usually well tolerated. Other oral agents and combination therapies are available through clinical trials. To learn more about the
possibility of participating in a clinical trial in your area, ask your
medical oncologist or neuro-oncologist.

Despite surgery, radiation, and chemotherapy, sometimes the
tumor continues to grow or, after a period of stability, begins to

grow again. After careful consideration and much discussion with the treatment team, the patient will choose either to undergo other forms of treatment or to decline further interventions. Indeed, some individuals decide they would rather travel or spend time with family than pursue aggressive medical treatments. There is no one right answer.

Chapter 10

Metastatic Brain Tumors

Martha is a vintage car enthusiast (she and her husband, Fred, own a '32 Ford Roadster), a crafter of pinecone wreaths, and has been working since age 16. Today, at 54 years old, she's on disability insurance for a quadruple whammy—breast cancer that metastasized to her lymph nodes, lungs, liver, and, ultimately, to her brain.

Martha has weathered a dizzying array of treatments and their side effects to arrest the spreading cancer. "The chemo [drugs] they use in the lower extremities do not break the blood–brain barrier to penetrate the brain," she says. So, when the cancer entered her brain in the form of four lesions, the devastation felt more than cumulative. "All I could think is my brain controls everything in my body," she says. "You don't know if you're going to go blind, lose your speech." Her first reaction, she says, was fear. "Things I can't control, I get scared of," she explains.

After aggressive treatment using whole-brain radiation and chemotherapy, Martha is relieved—for now—to report that two of the lesions are gone, and the other pair has shrunk by half. "I'm just waiting now," she says, for results from an upcoming computerized tomography (CT) scan. But she remains optimistic, no longer afraid to laugh at life's ironies. "I was planning on working towards retirement," she says. "Then, you find out at 50 years old, you're working to save your life.

"I have an Australian mesquite tree that I decorate with angels," she adds. "That's where I sit. I don't want the excitement of life to go away because I don't want to feel like I'm giving up."

Brain metastases (secondary brain tumors) are tumors that begin elsewhere in the body and travel to the brain. Lung cancer is the most common origin of this cancer type, followed by cancers of the breast, skin (melanoma), kidney (renal cell), and gastrointestinal region (colon and others). The number of patients whose cancer has traveled from areas within the body to the brain seems to be on the rise. This increase is likely the result of improvements in imaging techniques, such as magnetic resonance imaging (MRI), which are able to detect systemic cancers, as well as from improved therapies for cancer treatment. Individuals with certain cancers are now living longer than ever before; with that increased life span, the opportunity for cancers to spread to the brain has also increased, resulting in greater numbers of brain metastases being reported.

Systemic cancers can travel in many different vehicles on their journey to the brain. Cancer cells will ride through the bloodstream or lymphatic system, or they may penetrate the brain directly from the surrounding skull. Once cancer cells establish themselves within the brain, they invade the normal brain tissue and grow and divide in an uncontrolled manner, leading to the formation of a tumor. In brain metastases, it is common for multiple tumors to form within the brain, though solitary, or single, metastases can also occur (Figure 10–1A and Figure 10–1B).

Most people who experience brain metastases already know the nature and location of their primary cancer. Some, however, receive a dual diagnosis of systemic cancer and brain metastases all at once. For these individuals, lung cancer is the most frequent culprit. In rare cases, the original

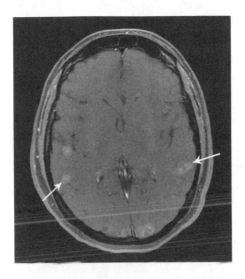

Figure 10–1A Brain metasteses 1.

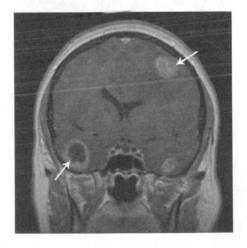

Figure 10–1B Brain metasteses 2.

source of cancer remains unknown; these cases are referred
to as "cancers of unknown primary site."

In this chapter, you will learn the following:

- **What a metastatic brain tumor is**
- **Where it typically comes from**
- **How it is diagnosed, and the symptoms**
- **The current best treatments**
- **How treatment differs for single and multiple
  metastases**
- **What leptomeningeal disease, or drop metastases, is and
  how it differs from metastatic brain tumors**

Symptoms

Metastases tend to grow quickly thanks to the nutrient-rich surroundings of brain tissue. The site in the brain in which a tumor, or
tumors, is growing will strongly determine a patient's symptoms.
Some people may report an unusual headache. Others may experience something as subtle as a blurring of the vision or something so
dramatic as a seizure, an abnormal increase in the electrical activity
of the brain that can lead to sensory symptoms, motor symptoms,
or generalized convulsions with loss of consciousness. Some may
feel weakness or numbness in either their arms or legs. Vexingly,
the signs may be as subtle as a minor personality change—an outgoing individual can become quiet and inward, or a person may just
seem confused—or they can be more severe, with the person having trouble with thinking and memory. Occasionally, elderly people
may be misdiagnosed with dementia or a stroke; only when an MRI
or CT scan is performed will the brain metastases be found. For
further details regarding the anatomy of the brain and possible
signs and symptoms of brain tumors, refer to Chapter 1.

Diagnosis

When an individual with a known cancer comes in for treatment, the physician will likely perform a battery of imaging tests in order to "stage" the disease. This means that the doctor is gathering information to understand the full extent to which the cancer has invaded the body and, possibly, the brain. During this step, an MRI or CT scan of the brain is frequently performed. For many people, these images will not reveal any evidence of spreading cancer. In others, however, the images will show that cancer has spread to the brain without having caused any neurologic symptoms.

Sometimes, an individual whose systemic cancer is in remission will later develop brain metastases. He or she may experience a neurologic symptom, prompting brain imaging, and find that the cancer has returned. In this example, the medical team will likely conduct another staging survey to assess the extent of the cancer. This staging can include multiple imaging and blood tests.

Treatment

Once the metastatic tumor is found on MRI, a patient may be given corticosteroids to reduce any irritation and swelling in the surrounding brain tissues. Easing the local irritation often reduces the symptoms—though, of course, it won't cure the tumor. At the same time, steroid use has its own side effects, including increased blood sugar, insomnia, behavioral changes, shaking and trembles, and stomach pain. For this reason, steroids are most often used as a short-term treatment. If steroids are needed for longer periods, the individual will be prescribed other medications to help protect against the development of osteoporosis, stomach ulcers, and diabetes.

In the event of a seizure resulting from brain metastases, a patient will likely be placed on an antiepileptic (antiseizure) medication. Several antiepileptic medications are commonly used in the oncology field, many of which do not interfere with chemotherapy.

Surgery

In rare cases, a person may be cured of one type of cancer only to develop brain metastases later. If the staging fails to reveal the original source, a tumor biopsy may need to be done to confirm the tissue diagnosis.

When a metastatic tumor is suspected, and it is located where it can be safely operated upon, a resection can be performed. This approach tends to be reserved for people with a single metastatic tumor who are in good enough health to tolerate brain surgery. After a successful surgical removal, most of these individuals enjoy a prolonged life.

Multiple Metastases

To relieve immediate symptoms, surgery may be appropriate for people with tumors in life-threatening areas of the brain. Otherwise, those with multiple metastases receive no clear survival benefit from brain surgery. For further details regarding the various surgical procedures, please refer to the surgical subsection of Chapter 9.

Radiation Therapy

Most people with a metastatic brain tumor end up receiving whole-brain radiation therapy (WBRT). WBRT is typically administered over 2 weeks and will likely be accompanied by surgery or chemotherapy. Stereotactic radiosurgery (SRS) is another method for delivering radiation to metastatic brain tumors. SRS is preferred when the individual has one to three tumors that measure less than 3 centimeters each. Occasionally, people with brain metastases are treated with both WBRT and SRS. Using both forms of radiation, however, increases the risk of permanent brain damage from radiation necrosis. For further details on radiation therapy and its potential risks and benefits, refer to Chapter 3.

Chemotherapy

The treatment of metastatic brain tumors can be frustrating, because the underlying systemic cancer that caused it must also be treated at the same time. This treatment often takes the form of chemotherapy, which fortunately also helps in treating brain metastases. A discussion of current chemotherapy treatments for various systemic cancers that can cause brain metastases is beyond the scope of this book. Please ask your oncologist for further information regarding resources and treatments for your specific tumor type.

A hardcore planner, Martha is preparing—for her wedding, and for her death. She is planning a celebration to renew her vows to her husband of 15 years, Fred, surrounded by 50 friends and family members. At the same time, she's teaching Fred to cook, pay the bills, and upload photos on e-mail. "These are things he's never had to do because he always had me to do it," she says. "I'm teaching him to take care of himself." Juggling a wedding and a funeral has kept Martha busy and engaged. "I've asked my minister to bury me and marry me," she says. "I need to write my vows. I want to get rid of 'till death do you part' and go with the 'eternity' thing."

Prognosis

Prognosis varies based on tumor type, the individual's age, general health, and performance status. Without any treatment, brain metastases may cause death in a matter of weeks to months, on average. With the use of WBRT, the average survival is often extended for several months. Survival greater than 1 year after original detection of brain metastases is rare but does happen. For further discussion regarding end-of-life care, please refer to Chapter 5.

Leptomeningeal Disease

Some tumors, most often breast cancer, lung cancer, and lymphoma, can also spread into the fluid surrounding the brain. This pattern of growth is called **leptomeningeal** because the tumor cells float in the spinal fluid surrounded by the thin, spidery covering over the brain, known as the meninges. Adhesive in nature, these tumor cells often stick to the surface of the brain, the cranial nerves, and the nerve roots in the arms and legs. As a result, they can produce unusual symptoms, such as asymmetric pain in one arm or leg or loss of vision in one eye.

Leptomeningeal disease is sometimes also called **drop metastases**. The term describes how certain brain tumors "drop" down the fluid of the thecal sac (a membrane that surrounds the spinal cord and circulates cerebral spinal fluid) and attach to nerve roots in a growth pattern that resembles a strand of pearls.

Treatment

Because they compete with nerves for nutrients, the tumor cells are treated through the direct injection of chemotherapy into the brain, either through a spinal tap or by using a specialized catheter called an **Ommaya reservoir** (Figure 10–2). This "transfer station" is surgically implanted under the scalp and attached via catheter to a ventricle. Upon its insertion, medicines can be administered directly to the brain through a small needle poke into the scalp. As a result, this method is considered to be an effective, less invasive

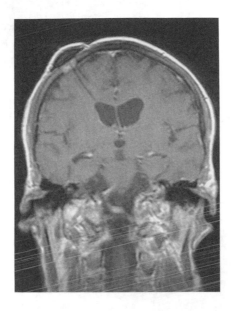

FIGURE 10-2 Front view of a brain showing an Ommaya reservoir in place in the right frontal lobe. Note the catheter can be seen ending in the fluid of the right lateral ventricle. The reservoir under the scalp fills with spinal fluid and can be accessed there by a small needle.

way to distribute the chemotherapy to the spinal fluid than when injected into the low back.

The chemotherapy agent selected by the physician is tailored to the patient's specific cancer type. Drugs like methotrexate and Ara-C are often used intrathecally (directly in the spinal fluid) and can be injected twice weekly. A lipid substance called cytarabine liposome, a sustained-release ara-c, can be infused every other week. Dexamethasone is often needed in higher doses to prevent the chemotherapy from inflaming the nerves and causing pain, and antinausea medication is also sometimes necessary.

At each treatment, the free-floating tumor cells can be measured. If the chemotherapy has proved effective, the patient can enter a maintenance phase designed to keep the cells from growing back.

Leptomeningeal type of tumor growth can also occur with some solid brain tumor types, especially those located in the posterior fossa around the cerebellum. Such tumors include medulloblastoma, pineoblastoma, and primitive neuroectodermal tumors. Because these tumors occur more frequently in children than in adults, a leptomeningeal growth pattern is more commonly seen in children.

Guide to Drugs Prescribed for
Brain Tumors

The following is a list of drugs discussed throughout the book that we hope will serve as a useful reference. The list contains the generic name for each drug followed by common brand names and a brief description of when and why it is used in the treatment of brain tumors.

Bevacizumab *(Avastin)*
   An intravenous monoclonal antibody administered twice monthly for use in recurrent glioblastoma.
Bisacodyl *(Alophen, Bisac-Evac, Bisco-Lax, Carter's Little Pills, Colax, Correct, Correctol, Dulcogen, Dulcolax, Evac-U-Gen, Ex-lax Ultra, Feen-A-Mint, Fematrol, Fleet Bisacodyl, Gen Lax, Gentlax, Modane, Veracolate, Doxidan)*
   Used on a short-term basis to treat constipation.
Bromocriptine *(Cycloset, Parlodel)*
   Used to treat symptoms of hyperprolactinemia (high levels of a natural substance called prolactin in the body) caused by certain types of tumors that produce prolactin, and it may shrink these tumors.
Cabergoline *(Dostinex, Cabaser)*
   Used to treat different types of medical problems that occur when too much of the hormone prolactin is produced.

Carbamazepine *(Carbatrol, Epitol, Equetro, Tegretol)*
Used alone or in combination with other medications to control certain types of seizures.
Carmustine *(BCNU)*
Used in the treatment of several types of brain cancer, including glioma, glioblastoma multiforme, medullobalstoma, and astrocytoma.
Coumadin *(Warfarin)*
Used to prevent blood clots from forming or growing larger in the blood and blood vessels.
Cyclophosphamide *(Cytoxan)*
Oral chemotherapy used alone or in combination with other medications to treat certain cancers by slowing or stopping the growth of cancer cells.
Cytarabine *("Ara-c") (Cytosar-U)*
Intravenous chemotherapy used to treat different forms of leukemia, meningeal leukemia and lymphoma (cancers found in the lining of the brain and spinal cord).
Dexamethasone *(Decadron, Dexasone, Diodex, Hexadrol, Maxidex)*
A strong oral corticosteroid medication that decreases brain swelling.
Diphenhydramine *(40 Winks, Aler-Dryl, Alka-Seltzer Plus Allergy, Allergia-C, Allermax, Altaryl, Antihist, Antituss, Banophen, Beldin, Belix, Ben Tann, Benadryl, Benekraft, Bromanate AF, Bydramine, Compoz, Correct Dose Childrens Allergy Relief, Dicopanol, Diphedryl, Diphen, Diphenadryl, Diphendryl, Diphenhist, Diphenmax, Diphenyl, Diphenylin, Dytan, Dytuss, Elixsure Allergy, Genahist, Hydramine, Kids-Eeze Allergy, Nervine, Nu-Med, Nytol, Pardryl, Paxidorm, PediaCare Children's Allergy, Pediacare Nighttime Cough, Rest Simply, Scot-Tussin Allergy, Siladryl, Siladyl, Silphen, Simply Sleep, Sleep-Eze, Sleep-ettes, Sleepinal, Sleeptabs, Sominex, Somnicaps, Theraflu Multi Symptom, Triaminic Cough & Runny Nose, Tusstat, Twilite, Uni-Hist, Uni-Tann, Unisom Sleep, Valu-Dryl, Wal-Dryl Allergy, Wal-Dryl Childrens, Wal-Som Maximum Strength, Zzzquil)*

Used to relieve red, irritated, itchy, watery eyes; sneezing; and runny nose caused by hay fever, allergies, or the common cold. Often used in conjunction with intravenous chemotherapy to improve tolerance and limit side effects.

Dolasetron *(Anzemet)*

Used to prevent nausea and vomiting caused by cancer chemotherapy, anesthesia, or surgery.

Doxorubicin *(Adriamycin PFS, Adriamycin RDF, Adriamycin, Doxil)*

An intravenous chemotherapy targeting cellular DNA.

Hydroxyurea *(Droxia)*

Used to treat skin cancer (melanoma), a cancer of the white blood cells called chronic myelocytic leukemia (CML), and metastatic cancer (cancer that has spread) of the ovaries. This medicine may also be given together with radiation treatment for head and neck cancer (primary squamous cell cancer).

Ibuprofen *(Addaprin, Advil, Cap-Profen, Counteract IB, Dolgesic, Genpril,*

Haltran, IB Pro, IBU-200, Ibifon 600, Ibren, Ibu, Ibu-Tab, Ibuprohm, Midol Cramps & Bodyaches, Menadol, Motrin, Nuprin, Q-Profen, Rufen, Rx-Act Ibuprofen, Saleto, Samson 8, Sup Pain Med, Tab-Profen, Ultraprin, Uni-Pro, Wal-Profen)

A nonsteroidal anti-inflammatory drug used to relieve pain, tenderness, swelling, and stiffness.

Ironotecan *(Camptosar)*

An intravenous chemotherapy drug targeting cellular DNA targeting cellular DNA.

Lamotrigine *(Lamictal)*

Extended-release tablets used with other medications to treat certain types of seizures

Levetiracetam *(Keppra)*

Used alone or in combination with other medications to treat certain types of seizures in people with epilepsy.

Lomustine *(CCNU, CeeNU)*
A highly lipid soluble oral chemotherapy drug able to cross the blood–brain barrier, making it useful for treating brain tumors.

Lorazepam *(Ativan)*
Used to treat nausea, anxiety, and to stop seizure activity.

Methotrexate *(Rheumatrex, Trexall)*
Used in IV form to treat CNS lymphoma and occasionally administered intrathecally to treat leptomeningeal metastases.

Methylphenidate *(Ritalin, Ritalin SR, Methylin, Methylin ER)*
Used as part of a treatment program to control symptoms of attention and fatigue, or to improve brain function in brain tumor patients.

Ondansetron *(Zofran)*
Used to prevent nausea and vomiting caused by cancer chemotherapy, radiation therapy, and surgery.

Oxycodone *(Dazidox, ETH-Oxydose, Endocodone, Oxecta, Oxy IR, Oxycontin, Oxyfast, Percolone, Roxicodone)*
Used to relieve moderate to severe pain.

Pentoxifylline *(Pentopak, Pentoxil, Trental)*
Used commonly to improve blood flow in patients with circulatory problems to reduce aching, cramping, and tiredness in the hands and feet. Used on an experimental basis for treating radiation necrosis.

Phenergan *(Promethazine)*
Used to combat nausea caused by chemotherapy.

Phenytoin *(Di-Phen, Dilantin, Phenytek)*
Used to control certain type of seizures and to treat and prevent seizures that may begin during or after surgery to the brain or nervous system.

Sildenafil *(Revatio, Viagra)*
Used to treat erectile dysfunction in men.

Sulfamethoxazole *(Gantanol, Bactrim, Septra, Sulfatrim)*
A double-strength antibiotic used primarily in combination
with trimethoprim, a combination product known as Bactrim
or Septra. May be given in addition to chemotherapy to prevent infection in the urinary and pulmonary systems.

Tadalafil *(Adcirca, Cialis)*
Used to treat erectile dysfunction in men and pulmonary arte-
rial hypertension.

Temozolomide *(Temodar, Temodal)*
An oral chemotherapy frequently prescribed in conjunction
with and after radiation therapy for Grade 3 and Grade 4
gliomas that works by disrupting the DNA of tumor cells.

Valproic acid *(Depakene, Depakote, Epilim, Stavzor)*
Used alone or with other medications to treat certain types of
seizures.

Vincristine *(Oncovin, Vincasar)*
A drug administered by injection used in cancer chemotherapy.

Sources

Chemocare.com

http://www.chemocare.com

Mayo Clinic

http://www.mayoclinic.com/health/drug-information/
drugherbindex

US National Library of Medicine's PubMed Health

http://www.ncbi.nlm.nih.gov/pubmedhealth
http://www.nlm.nih.gov/medlineplus/druginformation.html

GLOSSARY

Acoustic neuroma: A tumor that grows on the sheath surrounding the eighth cranial nerve.

Acromegaly: A condition resulting from a tumor of the pituitary gland in which an excessive amount of growth hormone can result in an enlarged forehead, lower jaw, hands, or feet.

Anaplastic: The change in cells toward a cancerous form; often used in combination with tumor type, for example, anaplastic oligodendroglioma, anaplastic astrocytoma, and anaplastic meningioma.

Anaplastic astrocytoma: A grade 3 astrocytoma, a common form of primary brain tumor that tends to grow aggressively and may cause neurologic symptoms in a rapid or sudden manner.

Angiogenesis: A tumor's ability to make and sustain its own blood vessels.

Angiogram: A test used to assess the blood vessels in the brain and, specifically, to study the blood supply to the tumor itself.

Aphasia: A difficulty with language, often resulting from left temporal-parietal lobe tumors within the speech center.

Aquaplastic mask: A mask made of a plastic mesh material used to immobilize the patient's head and face to determine the optimal head position during external beam radiation therapy.

Astrocytoma: One of the most common forms of primary brain tumor, named for its cells of origin, the star-shaped glial cell (astrocyte).

Benign: A tumor that tends to grow slowly and may not be associated with any symptoms. (See Grade 1.)

Biopsy: The surgical retrieval of a small portion of tumor tissue, usually performed for the diagnosis of a tumor in circumstances where the tumor is too large or too close to important brain structures for complete removal.

Brachytherapy: The surgical implantation of radiation energy into or near a tumor.

Brain tumor: A mass of cells that forms and grows within the skull; may be benign or malignant. (See Grades 1–4.)

Brainstem: The stalk upon which the cerebral hemispheres sit, connecting them to the spinal cord.

Burr hole: A small opening in the skull made with a specialized surgical drill.

Cellularity: The degree of density of cells contributing to the appearance of a tumor mass.

Central nervous system: The part of the nervous system that consists of the brain and spinal cord responsible for the transmission of sensory and motor impulses.

Cerebellum: The balance and coordination center, located in the rear of the brain.

Cerebral hemispheres: The two primary divisions of the brain, consisting of left and right hemispheres, which sit atop the brainstem.

Cerebrum: Another term for the cerebral hemispheres that emphasizes that this is a part of the brain separate from the cerebellum.

Chemotherapy: The treatment of disease using chemicals that kill cancerous cells.

Clinical trial: A research study that involves people and follows a formal protocol. Generally, an evaluation of a drug begins in small Phase I and II trials and, if successful, moves into large, nationwide Phase III trials.

- Phase I: Toxicity trial (Is it toxic to humans?)

- Phase II: Efficacy trial (Does it work against a particular disease?)
- Phase III: Standard of care trial (Is it better than the current standard of care?)

Computerized tomography (CT) or (CAT) computerized axial tomography scan: A type of X-ray that uses contrast dye to provide information about the brain and skull.

Conservator: An individual appointed to manage finances, assets, and income of an individual who is incapacitated (a protected person). A conservator is responsible to handle financial matters for the protected person.

Cranial nerves: Twelve pairs of nerves that regulate sight, smell, taste, speech, hearing, swallowing, chewing, nonverbal expressions, and head and neck movement.

Craniotomy: The surgical removal of a piece of the skull to access the brain.

Debulk: A surgical removal of a part of the visible tumor; also known as a partial resection.

Deep venous thrombosis: A blood clot that forms in the veins of the calf and thigh.

Diagnosis: The act of identifying a disease from its symptoms.

Diplopia: Double vision caused by the impairment of the third, fourth, or sixth cranial nerve.

Dosimetrist: An expert who designs radiation therapy treatment plans for cancer patients.

Drop attacks: The sudden loss of one's ability to stand often caused by high pressure inside the skull created by a brain tumor.

Drop metastases: A term that describes how certain brain tumors cells "drop" down the fluid of the thecal sac (a membrane that surrounds the spinal cord and circulates cerebral spinal fluid) and attaches to nerve roots in a growth pattern that resembles candle wax drippings.

Dysarthria: A slurred speech pattern caused by impairment of the tenth cranial nerve.

Dysphagia: Difficulty in swallowing caused by impairment of the tenth cranial nerve.

Electroencephalogram (EEG): A study that uses electrodes to assess the brain's tendency toward seizure.

Ependymoma: A tumor that comes from the ependymal cells, which line the fluid-filled spaces in the brain.

External beam radiation therapy: A treatment that directs multiple radiation beams to deliver the desired radiation dose to the tumor while avoiding the normal surrounding brain tissues or critical structures.

Extra-axial: A tumor located outside the central nervous system, but within the skull, such as meningiomas, acoustic neuromas or schwannomas, and pituitary tumors.

Frontal lobes: A region of the brain that houses personality and executive functioning, such as critical thinking and decision making.

Gamma Knife: A machine specially designed for radiosurgery that provides radiation treatment with pinpoint accuracy.

Genetic markers: Hereditary factors that provide information about tumor type and the likelihood of responding to certain treatments.

Glial cells: Nonneuronal cells that maintain homeostasis, form myelin, and provide support and protection for the brain's neurons.

Glioblastoma multiforme (GBM): The most invasive form of glial tumor.

Glioma: One of the most common forms of primary brain tumor, named for its cells of origin, the star-shaped glial cell (astrocyte).

Grade: The degree of severity of disease, with severity increasing by number. The grade reflects the degree of cellular differentiation and refers to how much the tumor cells resemble or differ from normal cells of the same tissue type:

- Grade 1: Well differentiated (low grade)
- Grade 2: Moderately differentiated (intermediate grade)

- Grade 3: Poorly differentiated or anaplastic (high grade)
- Grade 4: Undifferentiated (high grade)

Gray (Gy): An absorbed dose of radiation.

Gross total resection (GTR): The surgical removal of an entire tumor through a hole made in the skull.

Guardian: A person appointed for the purpose of managing the personal affairs of an individual who is incapacitated (a ward). A guardian is responsible for making personal decisions and meeting needs for medical care, nutrition, clothing, shelter, or safety.

Health care directive: A written document, often also referred to as an advance directive, in which an individual appoints someone (a health care agent) to make health care decisions in the event he or she is unable to make them independently and to give instructions regarding health care.

Hemangiopericytoma: A rare tumor that arises from fibrous cells similar to those of a meningioma.

Hemiparesis: Weakness, or partial paralysis, in an arm and/or a leg on the same side of the body.

Hemiplegia: A complete paralysis in an arm and/or a leg on the same side.

Hospice: A facility or program designed to provide a caring environment for the physical and emotional needs of people who are terminally ill and their caregivers.

Intensity-modulated radiation therapy (IMRT): An advanced mode of high-precision radiotherapy that uses computer-controlled radiation beam shapers in the linear accelerators to pinpoint radiation doses to a malignant tumor or specific areas within the tumor and to minimize the dose to surrounding tissues.

Intra-axial: A tumor that forms within the central nervous system, such as gliomas and metastatic brain tumors.

Intracranial pressure: Pressure exerted by the blood and brain volumes inside the skull.

Ionizing radiation: X-rays or gamma rays directed to the tumor site, to damage the cells' ability to multiply.

Irrevocable trust: A trust that may not be changed or terminated after it has been established. It is a separate taxable entity, requiring its own tax identification number.

KI-67 stain: A chemical test performed in pathology on tumor tissue to measure what percent of the cells are rapidly dividing. (See Mitoses and MIB-1.)

Leptomeningeal: Having to do with the leptomeninges, the two innermost layers of tissues that cover the brain and spinal cord. (See Meninges.)

Leptomeningeal metastases: A form of cancer that has spread from the original (primary) tumor to the leptomeninges.

Leptomeninges: The two innermost layers of tissues that cover the brain and spinal cord.

Linear accelerator (Linac): A machine that produces radiation used for radiotherapy; it may also be adapted for radiosurgery or intensity modulated radiation therapy (IMRT).

Living trust: A trust created during the grantor's lifetime. Also called an inter vivos trust.

Lobes: The four sections—frontal, parietal, temporal, and occipital—of the brain. (See Cerebral hemispheres.)

Lumbar puncture: A procedure to gather cells from within the spinal fluid space in the thecal sac. A needle is inserted between the bones in the low back to obtain fluid, which is analyzed for the presence of certain sugars and proteins, as well as cell counts. Also known as a spinal tap.

Magnetic resonance angiogram (MRA): A type of imaging that uses magnetic fields to assess the blood vessels in the brain.

Magnetic resonance imaging (MRI): A type of imaging that uses magnetic fields to take highly detailed three-dimensional images of the brain.

Magnetic resonance spectroscopy (MRS): A special magnetic resonance imaging technique to evaluate certain metabolites in tumor tissue in an attempt to separate growing tumor from an expanding mass that may be simply scar tissue.

Malignant: A tumor that tends to grow aggressively and may spread to surrounding tissues by direct invasion or through the bloodstream. (See Grades 3–4.)

Medical oncologist: An internal medicine doctor who has received special training in cancer and administers chemotherapies for treatment.

Medulla oblongata: The part of the brain located atop the spinal cord that contains the centers for controlling involuntary functions.

Medulloblastoma: A highly malignant primary brain tumor that usually originates in the cerebellum or posterior fossa.

Meninges: The thin, spidery layer of cells that cover the brain and spine. (See Leptomeningeal.)

Meningioma: A tumor arising from the cells that cover the brain and spine, called the meninges, that is often diagnosed by accident and typically benign.

Metastasis: A mass of cells that originates in the body then spreads through the bloodstream to the brain.

Metastatic: A type of tumor that results from a spread of cancerous cells from other organs outside the brain (such as breast or lung).

MIB-1: A chemical test performed in pathology on tumor tissue to measure what percent of the cells are rapidly dividing. (See Mitoses and KI-67.)

Midbrain: The middle of the three primary divisions of the human brain, between the forebrain and the hindbrain.

Mitoses: A process that takes place in the nucleus of a dividing cell that results in the creation of two nuclei. Each dividing cell is called a mitotic figure.

Myelin: A substance in the brain that helps transmit impulses between neurons.

Necrosis: The presence of dead tissue.

Needle biopsy: A procedure through which a tiny sample of the tumor tissue is obtained through a small opening in the skull. (See Burr hole.)

Neural: Of or relating to nerves or the central nervous system.

Neurilemmoma: A tumor on the nerve to the inner ear; also known as a vestibular schwannoma or neuroma.

Neurologic: Of or pertaining to the nervous system.

Neurologist: A doctor who specializes in diseases of the central and peripheral nervous system.

Neuroma: A tumor arising from a nerve.

Neuro-oncologist: A neurologist who has completed specialty training in diagnosis and treatment of cancers of the central and peripheral nervous systems.

Neuropathologist: A doctor who evaluates tumor tissue of the brain and central nervous system on a glass slide through a microscope, and also the reaction of those cells to special chemical markers to allow determination of tumor grade.

Neuroradiologist: A doctor who specializes in reading and interpreting the results of imaging tests of the brain and central nervous system.

Neurorehabilitation: Providers of rehabilitation services, that is, speech therapists, physical therapists, occupational therapists, neuropsychologists, and physiatrists (a doctor specializing in physical medicine and rehabilitation).

Neurosurgeon: A doctor who operates on the brain, spinal cord, and nerves.

Occipital lobes: A region of the brain that aids in visual interpretation.

Oligodendrocytes: Cells within the brain that make myelin.

Oligodendroglioma: A primary brain tumor formed by an abnormal growth of oligodendrocytes.

Ommaya reservoir: A "transfer station" implanted under the scalp and attached via a small flexible tube ending inside a ventricle of the brain that allows for medicines to be administered directly into the spinal fluid.

Palliative care: Measures to reduce the symptoms or side effects of illness or its treatment.

Parietal lobes: A region of the brain that enables the understanding of direction and aids in visual-spatial orientation.

Pathologist: A doctor who studies the reaction of cells to special chemical markers and determines the nature of tumors by evaluating cell shape and size.

Pathology: The study of disease in bodily tissue.

PCP prophylaxis: The practice of prescribing a sulfa antibiotic oral drug to prevent the development of *Pneumocystis jiroveci* (formerly called *Pneumocystis carinii*) (PCP) in persons receiving chemotherapy and radiation therapy.

Pituitary adenoma: A tumor that develops in the tissue of the pituitary gland.

Pituitary gland: A gland located within the skull but outside the brain that produces and regulates the balance of hormones.

Pneumocystis (carinii) jiroveci pneumonia (PCP): A type of pneumonia caused by *Pneumocystis carinii*, a fungus, that can develop as a result of a reduced white blood cell count caused by radiation and chemotherapy. (See PCP prophylaxis.)

Pons: A region in the brainstem containing nerve fibers controlling facial and eye movement and sensation as well as the central nerve cells of the acoustic nerve.

Positron emission tomography (PET): This three-dimensional imaging test of the whole body able to confirm the presence of cancerous tissue throughout the body and brain. A PET scan can also be performed on the brain only in order to differentiate between the metabolic changes of benign or malignant tumors or to differentiate active tumor from pseudoprogression.

Power of attorney: A written document in which an individual (the "principal") appoints another person (the "attorney-in-fact") to handle property or finances.

Primary brain tumor: A tumor whose cancerous cells originate in the brain.

Prognosis: The art of using medical diagnosis and statistical predictions to help doctors and their patients understand future life expectancy and quality of life.

Proton therapy: A form of radiation treatment that uses a proton particle instead of X-rays to kill brain tumor cells.

Psammoma bodies: Rounded collections of calcium within a tumor.

Pseudoprogression: The death of healthy tissue caused by radiation therapy; a side effect of radiation therapy given to kill cancer cells. (Also called radiation necrosis.)

Radiation necrosis: The death of healthy tissue caused by radiation therapy; a side effect of radiation therapy given to kill cancer cells. (Also called "treatment-related pseudoprogression.")

Radiation oncologist: A doctor who has received special training to administer radiation therapy to assist in the treatment of malignancies.

Radiation technician: An individual trained in performing the technical details of radiation therapy.

Radiation therapy: A treatment that uses high-energy X-rays or other types of ionizing radiation to prevent the division of cancer cells.

Radiologist: A doctor who specializes in reading and interpreting the results of imaging tests, such as CT or MRI scans.

Recurrence: A tumor that has grown back after being removed or stabilized, often in the same area as the original tumor or in another part of the brain or spinal cord.

Remission: A state in which the tumor cells stop multiplying; may be temporary or permanent.

Resection: The surgical removal of a tumor. A total resection means the removal of all visible tumor. A subtotal or partial resection means that some of the visible tumor remains.

Revocable trust: A type of trust normally used for property management purposes. Such a trust may be changed, revoked, or terminated at any time during the lifetime of an individual as long as he or she is competent. After death, a revocable trust becomes irrevocable.

Schwannoma: A benign tumor of nerve fibers composed of Schwann cells.

Secondary brain tumor: A tumor whose cancerous cells originate in organs outside of the brain, spreading to the brain through the blood supply (also called metastasis).

Seizure: An electrical interruption in normal brain functioning.

Single-photon emission computed tomography (SPECT): A study of the brain performed in the nuclear medicine department to evaluate the metabolic rate of tumors in an attempt to differentiate active tumor growth from pseudoprogression.

Spinal tap: A test to retrieve cells from within the spinal fluid space in the thecal sac. A needle is inserted between the bones in the low back to obtain fluid, which is analyzed for the presence of certain sugars and proteins, as well as cell counts. Also known as a lumbar puncture.

Stereotactic radiosurgery (SRS): A treatment for brain tumors that involves the precise delivery of a single, high dose of radiation in a 1-day session. It is minimally invasive and uses a 3-dimensional coordinates system to locate small targets inside the body.(See Gamma Knife and Linac.)

Stereotaxy: A minimally invasive form of surgical intervention that uses a three-dimensional coordinates system to locate small targets inside the body.

Steroid myopathy: A weakening of the skeletal muscle caused by the use of a steroid to reduce brain swelling.

Subtotal resection: The surgical removal of some, but not all, of a tumor. (See Debulk.)

Temporal lobes: A region of the brain that contains the main structures for thinking, memory, and language; also most prone to seizures. (See Lobes and Hemispheres.)

Testamentary trust: A trust created by the terms of the grantor's will.

Three-dimensional conformal radiation therapy (3D-CRT): The most common form of external beam radiation therapy used in treatment of primary brain tumors.

Tumor: An abnormal mass of cells; may be malignant or benign. (See Brain tumor and Grades.)

Tumor board: A group of tumor specialists that meets regularly to review specific patients diagnosed with brain tumors; most common at large medical centers.

Vascular proliferation: The development of new blood vessels in tumors used to grow and support themselves. (See Angiogenesis.)

Ventricle: Spaces within the cerebrum and cerebellum that produce spinal fluid.

Vestibular schwannoma: A tumor on the nerve to the inner ear; also known as a neurilemmoma or acoustic neuroma.

Virtual tumor board: A group of tumor specialists that meets via Internet to review specific patients diagnosed with brain tumors.

Visual field deficits. A difficulty with vision to the left or right side, often resulting from occipital lobe tumors, that may impede driving, reading, cycling, and other activities.

Whole-brain radiation therapy (WBRT): A treatment that focuses radiation on the entire brain; most often used in the treatment of multiple tumors.

Will: A set of written instructions outlining how an individual wishes to have assets distributed upon death.

X-ray: High-energy radiation that can penetrate body parts to provide pictures of body parts (e.g., chest X-ray).

ABOUT THE AUTHORS AND CONTRIBUTORS

Lynne P. Taylor, MD, is a Fellow of the American Academy of Neurology and Neuro-oncologist and Director of Palliative Care at Tufts Medical Center in Boston, Massachusetts. Dr. Taylor graduated from Washington University School of Medicine and received her residency training in Neurology at the University of Pennsylvania and fellowship training in Neuro-oncology at Memorial Sloan-Kettering Cancer Center in New York. She is an Associate Professor (pending) in the division of Hematology-Oncology at Tufts Medical Center.

Alyx B. Porter Umphrey, MD, is the Director of the Neuro-oncology program at Mayo Clinic Arizona. Dr. Porter received her BA from Spelman College and MD from Temple University School of Medicine. Her residency and fellowship training was completed at Mayo Clinic Graduate School of Medicine in Rochester, Minnesota. Dr. Porter is an Assistant Professor of Neurology and Internal Medicine.

Diane Richard is a Minneapolis-based reporter, radio producer, and writer. She graduated from Smith College, Northampton, Massachusetts, and earned a master's of journalism from the University of Missouri, Columbia. Her documentaries have aired on public radio stations nationwide, and her writing has been published throughout the Twin Cities.

About the Contributors

The following contributors provided content expertise throughout the book.

Laurie Hanson, JD, is a shareholder with Long, Reher & Hanson, PA, an elder law firm in Minneapolis established to represent individuals and family members who are aging and/or living with disabilities. Ms. Hanson concentrates her practice exclusively in the areas of disability planning. Ms. Hanson is a member of the National Academy of Elder Law Attorneys and the Special Needs Alliance, a national professional association of attorneys committed to helping individuals with disabilities, their families, and the professionals who represent them.

Nancy's experience includes 6 years of caring for her husband, Randy, who died of brain cancer in 2006. She spearheaded the first-ever Caregiver Support Group through Seattle's Virginia Mason Hospital and continues to help new caregivers. To fulfill a promise to her husband, she became a spokesperson for Initiative 1000 that legalized the Death with Dignity Act in Washington State. She has given numerous interviews for TV, radio, and newspaper, and she will be featured in an HBO documentary called *How to Die in Oregon* (2011) that focuses on the Death with Dignity Law in Oregon and Washington. She has been a public speaker at many political, religious, and medical group events addressing the needs of the dying. She is a volunteer for Compassion and Choices of Washington (http://www.compassionwa.org), the nonprofit organization that is a steward of the Death with Dignity Act. She is also an active volunteer for Providence Hospice of Seattle (http://www2.providence.org/kingcounty/facilities/providence-hospice-of-seattle/Pages/default.aspx) and is an ordained minister.

Charles Nussbaum, MD, is a board-certified neurosurgeon. He completed his training at the University of Rochester in 1990. He is currently section head of neurosurgery at the Virginia Mason Medical Center in Seattle, Washington, where he is also a member of the Neuro-oncology team. He is also Secretary-Treasurer of the

Western Neurosurgical Society. Dr. Nussbaum contributed information about the neurosurgical approach to brain tumors.

Astrid Pujari, MD, is a board-certified internist and credentialed medical herbalist with years of experience providing consultation about the safe and effective integration of conventional and alternative therapies. Dr. Pujari received her medical degree from Tufts University School of Medicine in Boston, Massachusetts. She completed her internship and residency training in internal medicine at the Scripps Clinic and Research Institute in La Jolla, California. She also completed didactic and clinical training to obtain a 4-year medical herbalist degree from the Royal College of Phytotherapy in London, England. After rigorous academic and clinical examinations she was certified by the National Institute of Herbal Medicine (NIMH), the leading professional licensing body in Europe and the American Herbalist Guild. Dr. Pujari runs the Pujari Center for Spiritually Centered and Integrative Medicine in Seattle, Washington, and is a consultant at the Virginia Mason Medical Center Cancer Institute.

Huong Pham, MD, is a board-certified radiation oncologist with a special interest in treating central nervous system (CNS) tumors, having completed a radiation oncology CNS tumor fellowship at University of California, San Francisco, in 1997. She was an assistant professor and co-director of the Gamma Knife radiosurgery program at Case Western Reserve University from 1997 to 2000 before joining Virginia Mason Medical Center in Seattle, Washington, in 2001. Currently, she is the section head of radiation oncology and an active member of the Neuro-oncology program at Virginia Mason.

Murray Sagsveen, JD, is currently the chief operating officer and general counsel of The GOD'S CHILD Project. Previously, he was the general counsel of the American Academy of Neurology, chief executive officer of a state department of health, the general counsel of a state medical association, a partner in a law firm, and a judge advocate and brigadier general in the Army National Guard.

The American Academy of Neurology

An association of more than 25,000 neurologists and neuroscience professionals, is dedicated to promoting the highest quality patient-centered neurologic care. A neurologist is a doctor with specialized training in diagnosing, treating, and managing disorders of the brain and nervous system such as Parkinson's disease, brain tumors, Alzheimer's disease, stroke, migraine, multiple sclerosis, and epilepsy.

For more information about the Academy and its resources for people with neurologic disorders, visit *AAN.com*. To sign up for a free subscription to *Neurology Now®*, the Academy's magazine for patients and caregivers, visit *NeurologyNow.com*.

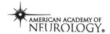

About the American Brain Foundation

The American Brain Foundation, the foundation of the American Academy of Neurology, is one of the largest providers of neurology research grants in the United States. The Foundation supports vital research and education to discover causes, improved treatments, and cures for brain and other nervous system diseases. Learn more at *CureBrainDisease.org*.

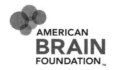

INDEX

abducens nerves, sixth cranial, 10, 11

accessory nerve, eleventh cranial, 10, 12

acoustic neuroma, 151–152, 153 radiation therapy, 57

acromegaly, pituitary adenomas, 149

Adriamycin, 147

advance directive, 114–115. *See also* health care directive

advanced registered nurse practitioners (ARNPs), 40

advocate, caregivers becoming, 101

Aging with Dignity, 136

alcohol consumption, 68

American Association of Brain Tumors, 75

American Bar Association, 136

American Brain Tumor Association, 36

anaplastic astrocytoma, 17, 61, 154, 162

angiogenesis (vascular proliferation), 165

angiogram, imaging, 28, 30

ankle-foot-orthosis (AFO), 88

Anzemet (dolasetron), 84

Aphasia, symptom, 87

Appointments, caregivers attending, 100–101

aquaplast mask, 48

Ara-C, 175

art, as therapy, 78, 79, 80

astrocytoma
anaplastic, 17, 61, 154, 162
cerebellar, 71, 101
chemotherapy, 164
driving with, 71–72
grade 4, 24, 164
primary brain tumor, 16, 17–18
types and grades, 161, 162

atomic bomb survivors, 20

attention deficit disorders, 55

authorized signer account, 120–121

automatic banking, 119

Avastin, 165

Bactrim, 85
bank accounts
    authorized signer account,
        120–121
    beneficiary designations, 121
    family caregiving contracts,
        122
    joint account, 120
    multiple-name, 119–122
    naming a representative
        payee, 121–122
    payable on death accounts,
        121
benign tumors, 15, 143
    acoustic neuroma, 151–152
    basics about meningioma,
        144–146
    life adjustments, 152–153
    pituitary adenoma, 148–151
    treating atypical and
        malignant meningiomas,
        146–148
    vestibular schwannomas, 151
bevacizumab, 165
biopsy, 25, 31, 35, 157–158
bisacodyl, 84
blood tests, 34–35
bone marrow biopsy, 35
brachytherapy, 47, 53
brain
    basics about, 8–13
    central nervous system (CNS),
        8–9
    computerized tomography
        (CT) image, 26
    cranial nerves and functions,
        10–12
    magnetic resonance imaging
        (MRI), 27

pituitary gland, 12
brain metastases, radiation
    therapy, 56
brainstem, 9, 10
brain swelling, side effect, 55
brain tumors
    astrocytoma, 16, 17–18
    average overall survival vs.
        percentage of long-term
        survivors, 44
    common primary, 15–19
    cure vs. progression-free
        survival, 43–44
    diagnosis, 3–4, 22–23
    ependymoma, 18–19
    expecting symptoms from,
        103
    glioblastoma multiforme
        (GBM), 14, 16, 17–18
    glioma, 17–18
    known and possible causes,
        20–22
    location, 14–15
    meningioma, 19
    oligodentroglioma, 17, 18
    pituitary tumor, 19
    retreatment, 56–57
    searching for causes, 20–22
    understanding, 13–19, 41–44
breathing deeply, 4, 65
bromocriptine, 150
burr hole, 157

cabergoline, 150
cancer
    brain tumors, 13–14
    possible dietary associations,
        21
cancer patient, label, 62

carbamazepine, 83
care arrangements, informal, 118
caregivers, 102–110
care team
  members, 38–40
  weighing options, 100
CaringBridge, 97
cellularity, 162
central nervous system (CNS), 8–9
cerebellar astrocytoma, 71, 101
cerebellar medulloblastoma, 90, 95
cerebellum, brain, 9, 10
cerebral hemispheres, brain, 9
change, caregivers embracing, 101–102
chemotherapy
  meningiomas, 147–148
  metastatic brain tumors, 173
  primary brain tumors, 164, 165–166
chronic fatigue, symptom, 86
Cialis, 91
Classifications, brain tumors, 13–15
clinical trials, primary brain tumors, 164–165
clinical trial staff, care team, 38
cognitive changes, symptom, 86–87
communication network, caregivers, 97
computer folder, collecting information, 45
computerized axial tomography (CT or CAT) scan
  imaging, 25, 26–27

conservator, 137
conservatorship, 136–138
constipation, symptom, 84
contrast agent, imaging, 31
cosmetic issues, 76–78
cranial nerves, 12 pairs and functions, 10–12
craniotomy
  scar, 77
  surgery, 32, 158
creativity, as therapy, 78, 79, 80
cyclophosphamide, 147
cytarabine liposome, 175

death, preparing for, 111
death and dying, 93
Death with Dignity initiative, 92, 95
debulked, 158
Decadron (dexamethasone), 82, 84, 89
deep venous thrombosis, symptom, 85
Department of Motor Vehicles (DMV), state laws, 72
Departments of Health, 136
Depression, symptom, 88–89
dexamethasone (Decadron), 82, 84, 89
diagnosis of brain tumor, 3–4, 22–23
  assembling your team, 6–7, 37–40
  assessment and plan, 25–35
  doctor's office, 5
  getting medical help, 35–36
  imaging techniques, 26–32
  Internet, 5–6
  keeping a journal, 7

diagnosis of brain tumor
    (*Cont'd*)
  metastatic brain tumors, 171
  second opinions, 5, 36–37
  seeking out information,
    4–6
  supplemental testing, 32–35
  support groups, 6, 75, 76
  survival, 43–44
  taking a deep breath, 4, 65
  taking charge, 44–45
  understanding prognosis,
    41–44
diet, healthy eating, 67–68
dietary associations, possible, to
    cancer, 21
dietary supplements, 69–71
diplopia, 11
direct deposit banking, 119
DNR/DNI/DNH (do not
    resuscitate/do not intubate/
    do not hospitalize), 135
doctor's office, brain tumor
    information, 5
dolasetron (Anzemet), 84
dosage, radiation therapy, 51
dosimetrists, 47
double vision, 11
doxorubicin, 147
driving, brain tumor patients,
    71–74
drop attacks, symptom, 82
drop metastases, leptomeningeal
    disease, 174–176
dry mouth, symptom, 86
dry test run, three-dimensional
    conformal radiation therapy
    (3D-CRT), 50
dura, 9

durable power of attorney,
    114–115, 122–125
dural tail, meningioma, 144

electroencephalogram (EEG),
    imaging, 31
emergency information. *See also*
    future planning
  caregivers, 108
  emergency notebook, 115–117
  planning, 114–115
emotional health, stress
    reduction, 63–64
emotions, 4
empowerment, brain tumor
    diagnosis, 62–63
ependymoma, primary brain
    tumor, 18–19
etiology, cause, 14
eulogies, caregivers sharing,
    before death, 112
exercise
  cancer patient, 66–67, 89
  caregivers staying active,
    106
external beam radiation therapy,
    47, 52–53
extra-axial, brain tumor, 13

facial nerve, seventh cranial, 10,
    11
faith, spirituality, 91–92
Family and Medical Leave Act
    (FMLA), 74–75
family caregiving contracts, 122
fatigue, symptom, 86
financial management
  authorized signer account,
    120–121

automatic banking and direct deposit, 119
beneficiary designations, 121
family caregiving contracts, 122
joint account, 120
multiple-name bank accounts, 119–122
naming a representative payee, 121–122
payable on death accounts, 121
first-party special needs trust, 129–130
fish oil, 70
frontal lobe, brain, 9
fun
  caregivers helping patient find, 108–109
  caregivers planning, 98
future planning
  authorized signer account, 120–121
  automatic banking and direct deposit, 119
  beneficiary designations, 121
  conservatorship, 136–138
  durable power of attorney, 114–115, 122–125
  emergencies, 114–115
  emergency notebook, 115–117
  family caregiving contracts, 122
  formal financial management services, 119–122
  guardianship, 136–138
  health care directives, 131–136

informal care arrangements, 118
joint account, 120
multiple-name bank accounts, 119–122
naming representative payee, 121–122
payable on death accounts, 121
Physician Orders for Life-Sustaining Treatment (POLST), 135–136
trusts, 125–131
will, 138–139

Gamma Knife procedure, 46, 52–53, 57
genetic markers, pathology report, 162 163
genetic syndromes, tumor development, 21
glioblastoma
  magnetic resonance imaging (MRI), 28, 29
  recurrent, 165
glioblastoma multiforme (GBM)
  primary brain tumor, 16, 17, 161
  temozolomide (Temodar), 51, 164
gliomas
  chemotherapy, 164
  primary brain tumor, 17–18
  recurrent, 52
  types and grades, 161
glossopharyngeal nerve, ninth cranial, 10, 12
green tea, 70–71

gross total resection, procedure, 31–32
guardian, 136
guardianship, 136–138
guided imagery meditation, 66

hair loss, 53–54, 76–77
hair prosthesis, 77
headache, symptom, 82
healing, caregiver and patient, 113
health care directive
    do not resuscitate/do not intubate/do not hospitalize (DNR/DNI/DNH), 135
    forms for, 136
    Physician Orders for Life-Sustaining Treatment (POLST), 135–136
health care directives, 131–136
    availability, 134
    cancelling or revoking, 134
    health care agent, 132, 133–134
    inclusions, 132–133
    Uniform Anatomical Gift Act, 134–135
healthful diet, 67–68
Health Insurance Portability and Accountability Act (HIPAA), 133
Hemiparesis, symptom, 88
herbal supplements, 69–71
hereditary factors, brain tumor, 22
hereditary non-polyposis colon cancer, 21
home preparation, caregivers, 105

hospice, 92, 111
human immunodeficiency virus (HIV), testing for, 35
humor, as therapy, 78, 80
hydrocodone, headache, 82
hydroxyurea, 147
hypoglossal nerve, twelfth cranial, 10, 12

ibuprofen, 82
imaging techniques
    angiogram, 28, 30
    computerized axial tomography (CT or CAT) scan, 25, 26–27
    gross total resection, 31–32
    magnetic resonance angiogram (MRA), 30–31
    magnetic resonance imaging (MRI), 25, 27–28
    magnetic resonance spectroscopy (MRS), 31, 32
    positron emission tomography (PET), 31, 32–33
    single-photon emission-computed tomography (SPECT), 31
    X-rays, 28
information
    brain tumor, 4–6
    caregivers gathering, 96–97
    emergency notebook, 115–117
    organizing in chronological order, 45
intensity-modulated radiation therapy (IMRT), external beam, 52, 57

Internet
  health care directive forms,
    136
  information, 5–6
  support groups, 75
intra-axial, brain tumor, 13
intracranial pressure, headache,
    82
ionizing radiation, 46
irrevocable trust, 126

joint account, banking, 120
journaling, 7, 78

KI-67 stain, 162

lamotrigine, 83
language difficulty, 87
laughing, caregivers, 98
leptomeningeal disease
  drop metastases, 174
  Ommaya reservoir, 174, 175
  treatment, 174–176
levetiracetam, 83
lifestyle management
  alcohol, 68
  breathing deeply, 65
  cosmetic issues, 76–78
  creativity, art and humor as
    therapy, 78, 80
  driving, 71–74
  empowerment, 62–63
  herbal and dietary
    supplements, 69–71
  meditation, 65–66
  nutrition, 67–68
  physical activity, 66–67
  quilting, 78, 79
  sleep, 64

stress reduction, 63–65
support groups, 75, 76
working, 74–75
Li-Fraumeni cancer syndrome,
    21, 163
limitations
  caregivers accepting, 104–105
  caregivers accepting new,
    106–107
linear accelerator, 47
living trust. *See also* trusts
  creating, 127–128
  defined, 125–126
lobes, brain, 9–10
location, brain tumors, 14–15
lorazepam, 84
love, caregiver and patient, 112
loved one's wishes, caregiver
    accepting, 110
lumbar puncture (spinal tap),
    33–34
lymphoma, 13
Lynch syndrome, 21

magnetic resonance angiogram
    (MRA), technique, 30–31
magnetic resonance imaging
    (MRI)
  glioblastoma, 28, 29
  imaging, 25, 27–28, 168, 169
  oligodedroglioma, 30
  radiotherapy, 46
magnetic resonance
    spectroscopy (MRS),
    imaging, 31, 32, 33, 34
maintenance people, team,
    104
makeup, applying, 77–78
malignant tumors, 15

meaning, caregivers helping patient find, 108–109
Medicaid, 96, 128–131
medical decisions, caregiver helping, 96
medical disability, 74–75
medical help, brain tumor, 35–36
medical oncologists
  care team, 38–39
  medical team, 7, 38
medical physicists, radiation oncology team, 47
Medicare, 96, 109
meditation, 65–66
medulla oblongata, brain, 9, 10
memorial service, caregiving helping loved one plan, 111
Memorial Sloan-Kettering Cancer Center, 70
meninges, 9
meningiomas
  axial view of brain, 145
  basics about, 144–146
  computerized tomography (CT), 144, 145
  magnetic resonance imaging (MRI), 145
  primary brain tumor, 19
  radiation therapy, 57
  treating atypical and malignant, 146–148
mental health, stress reduction, 64
metastasis, 25
metastatic brain tumors
  brain metastases, 168–170
  chemotherapy, 173
  classification, 13

diagnosis, 171
leptomeningeal disease, 174–176
multiple metastases, 172
prognosis, 173–174
prognostic indicators, 42
radiation therapy, 172–173
surgery, 172
symptoms, 170
treatment, 171–173
methotrexate, 175
methylguanine-DNA methyltransferase (MGMT), 163
methylphenidate, 55
MIB-index (Ki-67), 162
midbrain, 9, 10
mindfulness meditation, 66
mitoses, 162
multivitamins, 70
myopathy, steroid, 89

narcotics, headache, 82
National Brain Tumor Society, 15, 36, 75
National Cancer Institute, 36
National Hospice and Palliative Care Organization, 136
nausea, symptom, 84
navigation, 159
necrosis, 162
needle biopsy, 157
neurofibromatosis 2 (NF-2), 21, 151
neurologic progression-free survival, 43
neurologist, 6
neuro-oncologist, 6, 26, 100
neuropathologist. 39

neuroradiologist. 40
neurorehabilitation, 39
neurosurgeon, 6
    angiogram, 30
    care team, 39
    choosing, 156
    medical team, 38
notebook
    collecting information, 45
    emergency, 115–117
nutrition, 67–68
nutritionists, 47

occipital lobe, brain, 9–10
occupational therapists, driving
    screen, 73
oculomotor nerves, third cranial,
    10, 11
olfactory nerves, first cranial,
    10, 11
oligoastrocytoma
    types and grades, 161
oligodendroglioma
    magnetic resonance imaging
        (MRI), 30
    primary brain tumor, 17, 18
    types and grades, 161, 162
omega-3 oils, 70
omega-6 oils, 70
Ommaya reservoir, treatment,
    174, 175
ondansetron (Zofran), 84
optic nerves, second cranial, 10,
    11
oxycodone, headache, 82

palliative care, 81
Paradise Lost, Milton, 3
parietal lobe, brain, 9–10

partial paralysis, symptom, 88
pathologist, 39
pathology, 37
pathology report,
    understanding, 161–163
patient's goals, caregiver
    clarifying, 110
patient's return to work,
    caregivers helping, 99
payable on death (POD)
    accounts, 121
pergolide, 150
Phenergan, 84
phenytoin, 83
physical activity
    cancer patients, 66–67, 89
    caregivers, 106
Physician Orders for Life-
    Sustaining Treatment
    (POLST), 135–136
pituitary adenoma
    acromegaly, 149
    diagnosis, 149
    functioning and
        nonfunctioning,
        149–150
    imaging, 148
    radiation therapy, 57
    surgery, 150–151
    treatment paths, 150–151,
        153
pituitary gland, 12, 55
pituitary tumor, 19. *See also*
    pituitary adenoma
planning. *See* future planning
Pneumocystic jiroveci, 85
Pneumocystis carinii (PCP), 85
pons, brain, 9, 10
pooled trust, 131

positron emission tomography
    (PET), imaging, 31, 32–33
power of attorney. *See also*
    durable power of attorney
    cancelling or ending,
        124–125
    care in choosing attorney-in-
        fact, 123
    creating, 124
    defined, 123
    safeguards, 124
prescription medications,
    caregivers reading, 106
pre-surgery. *See* caregivers
primary brain tumors
    astrocytoma, 16, 17–18, 61,
        154
    biopsy, 157–158
    burr hole, 157
    chemotherapy, 164, 165–166
    classification, 13
    clinical trials, 164–165
    ependymoma, 18–19
    glioblastoma multiforme
        (GBM), 16, 17
    glioma, 17–18
    meningioma, 19
    needle biopsy, 157
    oligodendroglioma, 18
    pituitary tumor, 19
    prognostic indicators, 42
    radiation therapy, 163,
        165–166
    resection, 158–159
    subtotal resection, 159
    surgery, 156–161
    three-dimensional conformal
        radiation therapy (3D-CRT),
        48–50

understanding pathology
    report, 161–163
understanding treatment
    options, 155–161
prognosis
    metastatic brain tumors,
        173–174
    understanding, 41–44
progression-free survival, cure
    vs., 43–44
prolactinoma, 150
proton therapy, external beam,
    53
psammoma bodies, meningioma,
    144–145

quality of life
    caregiver, 94
    palliative care, 81
quilting, 78, 79

radiation necrosis, 55, 147
radiation oncologist, 7, 39–40
radiation oncology nurses, 47
radiation oncology team,
    members, 47–50
radiation technician, 40
radiation therapists, 47
radiation therapy
    acoustic neuroma, 57, 152
    brain metastases, 56
    brain tumors, 20–21
    considerations, 50–53
    dosage specifics, 51
    external beam radiation
        therapies, 47, 52–53
    Gamma Knife, 52–53
    intensity-modulated radiation
        therapy (IMRT), 52

meningioma, 57
metastatic brain tumors,
172–173
pituitary adenoma, 57
primary brain tumors, 46–47,
163, 165–166
proton therapy, 53
retreatment, 56–57
side effects, 53–55
stereotactic radiosurgery
(SRS), 52
stereotactic radiotherapy
(SRT), 52
radiologist, 40
angiogram, 30
radiotherapy, 46–47
rash, symptom, 90
reading, 88
recurrent gliomas, 52
registered nurses (RNs), 40
religion, spirituality, 91–92
Representative Payee Program,
121
resection, 158–159
rest, caregivers encouraging, 107
resveratrol, 71
retreatment, radiation therapy,
56–57
revocable trust, 126, 128
Ritalin, 55
rituals, caregivers creating, 106
routines, caregivers developing
new, 107

secondary brain tumors. *See also*
metastatic brain tumors
brain metastases, 168
classification, 13
prognostic indicators, 42

second opinions, brain tumor, 5,
36–37
seizures
brain metastases, 171–172
driving, 72–73
symptom, 82–84
senna, 84
sexuality, 90–91
side effects
caregivers expecting, from
treatments, 102
radiation therapy, 53–55
sildenafil, 91
single-photon emission-
computed tomography
(SPECT), imaging, 31, 32
skull, 13
sleep, recommendations, 64
Social Security, 96, 119, 121
social worker, 40, 47
Society for Neuro-Oncology, 36
specialists, brain tumor, 6–7
speech, aphasia, 87
spinal tap (lumbar puncture),
33–34
spiritual health, stress reduction,
65
spirituality, 91–92
status epilepticus, 84
stereotactic radiosurgery (SRS),
147
external beam, 52, 57
metastatic brain tumors,
172–173
stereotactic radiotherapy (SRT),
52, 57
stereotaxy, 159
steroid myopathy, 89
steroids, radiation necrosis, 55

stimuli, caregivers limiting, 108
stress reduction, 63–65
subtotal resection, 159
sulfamethoxazole, 85
Supplemental Security Income, 121
supplements, herbal and dietary, 69–71
supporters
    caregiver and patient, 113
    caregivers identifying core, 103–104
support groups
    brain tumors, 6, 75, 76
    caregivers joining, 99
surgery
    craniotomy, 32, 158
    metastatic brain tumors, 172
    pituitary adenomas, 150–151
    primary brain tumors, 156–161
survival
    average overall survival vs. percentage of long-term survivors, 44
    cure vs. progression-free, 43–44
    factors for long-term, 155
    statistics, 42–43
symptoms
    aphasia, 87
    caregivers expecting, from brain tumor, 103
    changes in taste, 86
    cognitive changes, 86–87
    constipation, 84
    deep venous thrombosis, 85
    depression, 88–89
    drop attacks, 82
    fatigue, 86
    headache, 82
    hemiparesis, 88
    metastatic brain tumors, 170
    nausea and vomiting, 84
    PCP prophylaxis, 85
    rash, 90
    reading, 88
    seizures, 82–84
    steroid myopathy, 89
    visual field deficits, 87–88

tadalafil, 91
taste changes, symptom, 86
team
    assembling specialists, 6–7, 37–40
    finalizing treatment, 41
temozolomide (Temodar), chemotherapy, 51, 84, 164
temporal lobe, brain, 9–10
therapy, creativity, art and humor, 78–80
third-party special needs trust, 130–131
three-dimensional conformal radiation therapy (3D-CRT), 48–50
transcendental meditation, 66
transportation, caregivers, 105
treatment. *See also* caregivers during treatment
    choosing neurosurgeon, 156
    leptomeningeal disease, 174–176
    meningiomas, 146–148
    metastatic brain tumors, 171–173
    pituitary adenoma, 150–151

pituitary adenomas, 150–151
primary brain tumors,
    155–161
weighing options, 100
trigeminal nerves, fifth cranial,
    10, 11
trochlear nerves, fourth cranial,
    10, 11
trusts
    basic living trust, 125–126
    care in choosing trustee,
        126–127
    creating living trust, 127–128
    first-party special needs,
        129–130
    irrevocable, 126
    living trust, 125
    pooled, 131
    protecting assets while
        dependent on Medicaid,
        128–131
    revocable, 126, 128
    testamentary trust, 125
    third-party special needs,
        130–131
tumor boards, 36–37
tumor markers, blood tests,
    34–35
turmeric, 71

Uniform Anatomical Gift Act,
    134–135
United States Pharmacopeia
    (USP), 69
U.S. Department of Veterans
    Affairs, 121
U.S. Food and Drug Administration
    (FDA), 69, 165
U.S. Living Wills Registry, 136

U.S. Office of Personnel
    Management, 121
U.S. Railroad Retirement Board,
    121

vagus nerve, tenth cranial, 10,
    12
valproic acid, 83
vascular proliferation
    (angiogenesis), 162
vestibular schwannomas,
    151–152
vestibulocochlear nerve, eight
    cranial, 10, 11
Viagra, 91
vincristine, 147
Virginia Mason Medical Center,
    Brain Tumor Support
    Group, 76
virtual tumor boards, 37
visual field deficits, symptom,
    87–88
visual field examination, 35
vitamin D, 70
vomiting, symptom, 84
von Hippel-Lindau syndrome, 21

Washington State, Death with
    Dying initiative, 92, 95
whole-brain radiotherapy (WBRT),
    56, 167, 172–173, 174
wills, 138–139
working, 74–75, 99

X-rays
    imaging, 28
    radiotherapy, 46

Zofran, 84